200 SHORT CASES IN CLINICAL MEDICINE

200 SHORT CASES IN CLINICAL MEDICINE

R. R. BALIGA MBBS, MD, DNB, MRCP(UK)

Departments of Cardiology
Royal Postgraduate Medical School
Hammersmith and Ealing Hospitals
University of London
London
UK

Formerly: Clinical Tutor, University of Aberdeen, Aberdeen, UK

Foreword by Professor H. A. Lee

Baillière Tindall
London Philadelphia Toronto Sydney Tokyo

Baillière Tindall
W. B. Saunders
24–28 Oval Road, London NW1 7DX, UK

The Curtis Center, Independence Square West
Philadelphia, PA 19106–3399, USA

55 Horner Avenue
Toronto, Ontario M8Z 4X6, Canada

Harcourt Brace & Company, Australia
30–52 Smidmore Street, Marrickville, NSW 2204, Australia

Harcourt Brace & Company, Japan
Ichibancho Central Building, 22–1
Ichibancho, Chiyoda-ku, Tokyo 102, Japan

First published 1993
Third printing 1995

A CIP record for this book is available from the British Library

ISBN 0–7020–1684–5

Typeset by Phoenix Photosetting, Chatham, Kent
Printed and bound in Great Britain by
Mackays of Chatham PLC, Chatham, Kent

CONTENTS

RESPIRATORY SYSTEM

ABDOMEN

RHEUMATOLOGY

ENDOCRINOLOGY

DERMATOLOGY

MISCELLANEOUS

FOREWORD

Taking the final medical examinations or, indeed, Membership is one of those necessary milestones for any aspiring doctor and, with respect to Membership, for those wishing to continue, particularly, in hospital practice. There can be no doubt that many doctors fail the second part of the Membership because they are ill prepared and should not have been allowed to take the examination. However, on the other hand, there are a number of well-informed, experienced doctors who, when they come to examination fall apart because they cannot simultaneously think about the clinical signs and their implications which would have bearing on any subsequent discussions with the examiner. The short case section of the Membership is known to be the most discriminating part of the examination and is therefore by definition the most demanding.

Clearly, to pass the clinical part of the final MB or Membership examination the individual must be well prepared. This means that he or she will have seen many cases, often similar, in many different settings, and will have learnt how to integrate clinical findings with any other known data (e.g. family history, investigations), so as to come to a reasonable conclusion concerning the condition, treatment and prognosis. Certainly, the candidate is expected to localise the system at fault and to appreciate the consequences of the disease problem that he or she is examining in any subsequent discussions. He or she must be aware of the appropriate investigations to ask for and the important differential diagnoses. The candidate must present his or her findings logically and discuss the case in a comprehensive, sensible manner, not darting from one train of thought to another and clutching at straws.

The short cases examination does not involve looking at rarities. Most of the cases will present at many different hospitals on many occasions, with very similar signs and symptoms. The examinations are not designed to 'catch people out' but to determine those who really are competent to go on to higher things.

Nevertheless, because of the difficulties encountered by some well-informed students and experienced doctors, it is always useful to have some form of guideline, strategy, or even an aide-mémoire that might help them present their findings and proceed to discussions in a more coherent, logical way. This book is designed to do just that. The contents presented are not the result of simply collecting 200 cases, putting them together and letting the unfortunate reader decide for him- or herself. The material presented herein is a true reflection of what goes on in Finals and the Membership examinations. The cases have been selected because they represent the rump of the cases seen in examinations, not the rarities. The model answers given are not to be remembered parrot fashion but to be understood in terms of how they address the issues raised by the signs detected by the examinee.

There will always be candidates who, no matter how many courses they go to, however many different patients they see, will have some of the difficulties referred to above. It is my view therefore, that this carefully presented collection of cases and the style of the model answers given will help these candidates. It has been my pleasure to read through the draft phases of this book and I am confident that this final presentation will be warmly received by future cohorts of examinees.

Professor HA Lee BSc (Hons) MBBS (Hons) FRCP MRCS
Director of Wessex Regional Renal and Transplant Unit
Consultant General Physician to Portsmouth Group of Hospitals

PREFACE

This book has one aim above all others and that is to provide strategies to satisfy the requirements of a clinical examination in general medicine. Clinical examination is passed not solely on the breadth of theoretical knowledge but also on the masterly application of clinical skills and strategies. Practice at the bedside is the key to success and this book provides the required strategies to cope with the examination situation. Each candidate will have to mix and match these strategies depending on a given examination situation.

In writing this book I have assumed that readers will have a background knowledge of general medicine and will frequently consult textbooks of medicine and books on clinical methods. It does not serve to replace textbooks of medicine, books on clinical methods or bedside clinical examination.

Salient features of the book include the following:

● 200 short cases (not including the schemes provided for examination of each system) are arranged in the frequency they are seen in the ward and consequently the clinical examination.
● Almost all chapters begin with a suggested scheme for the examination of that particular system.
● Cases which are seen commonly in the ward and the clinical examination are discussed in greater detail than others.
● Cases for examinations are drawn from the same pool for both undergraduate and postgraduate examinations, although in the latter the candidates' performance has to be faultless and will be expected to know certain aspects in greater detail.

Each short case is discussed under the following headings:

● **Instruction.** This allows the candidate to know what sort of instruction or command he may expect from an examiner.
● **Salient features.** This section highlights the important features in each case and provides guidelines concerning what else the candidate has to look for in a given case and what to tell the examiner in order to satisfy the examiner that the candidate is 'safe and sound' to be a junior doctor.

• **Questions.** This section supplies the questions – with answers – which a candidate can expect in a given case. It also tends to serve as a 'minibook of lists' relevant to a clinical examination. A solid box (■) and a change of typeface demarcates questions which are of interest to the postgraduate, enabling undergraduates to concentrate on easier questions. After the questions there may be a brief list of major contributors relevant to that particular case; some examiners enjoy asking candidates about these.

• **References.** The list of references provided will be invaluable for the senior medical student, postgraduate and house officer.

I believe that this handbook will meet the needs of medical students and remove some of the fears naturally felt before examinations. This book is also useful for PLAB examination. I encourage your comments and opinions.

I thank Professor HA Lee for writing the Foreword and my wife Jay for doing my share of the domestic chores while I worked on this book. I thank Dr Steve Handley of Baillière Tindall for his support. I also thank Mr Nigel Eyre for his excellent job in editing this book.

RRB
London

Dedicated to
Professor Sir Stanley Peart FRS
and my parents
Ramakrishna and Shanthi Baliga
for their guidance

ACKNOWLEDGEMENTS

I wish to thank the following for their support.

In Aberdeen
Prof. JC Petrie FRCP, Dr J Webster FRCP, Dr TA Jeffers FRCP, Dr N Benjamin MRCP, Dr K McHardy MRCP (Department of Medicine and Therapeutics)
Dr AW Hutcheon FRCP, Dr DJ King MRCP (Department of Clinical Oncology)
Dr MJ Williams FRCP, Dr LE Murchison FRCP (Department of Diabetes and Endocrinology)
Dr PW Brunt FRCP, Dr NAG Mowat FRCP, Dr TS Sinclair FRCP, Dr A McKinley MRCP (Department of Gastroenterology)

In London
Dr J Kooner MD, MRCP (Royal Postgraduate School of Medicine, Hammersmith and Ealing Hospitals)
Dr M Jacyna MD, MRCP (Northwick Park Hospital)
Prof. H Thomas FRCP, Prof. D Sheridan FRCP, Prof. CJ Mathias FRCP, Dr W Sunman MRCP, Dr A Saini MRCP (St Mary's Hospital Medical School)

In Portsmouth
Prof. HA Lee FRCP, Dr Venkat Raman MRCP

In Stoke Mandeville
Dr HL Frankel FRCP, Mr I Nuseibeh FRCS and Dr DJ Short MRCP

In Leeds
Dr PV Bhandary, Dr L Bhandary

In Windsor and Slough
Mr PO Watts FRCS, Dr T Viegas

CARDIOVASCULAR SYSTEM

Examination of the Cardiovascular System

1. Introduce yourself: 'I am Dr/Mr/Ms .... May I examine your heart?'.

2. Ensure adequate exposure of the precordium: 'Would you pop your top things off, please'. However, be sensitive of the feelings of female patients.

3. Get the patient to sit at 45 degrees – use pillows to support the neck.

4. Inspection: comment on the patient's decubitus (whether he or she is comfortable at rest or obviously short of breath); comment on malar flush (seen in mitral stenosis).

5. Examine the pulse: rate (count for 15 s), rhythm, character, volume; lift the arm to feel for the collapsing pulse. Feel the other radial pulse simultaneously.

6. Comment on the scar at antecubital fossa (cardiac catheterisation scars).

7. Look at the tongue for pallor, central cyanosis.

8. Look at the eye for pallor, Argyll Robertson pupil.

9. Examine the jugular venous pulse: comment on the wave form and height from the sternal angle. Check abdominojugular reflux.

10. Comment on any carotid pulsations (Corrigan's sign of aortic regurgitation).

11. Examine the precordium: comment on surgical scars (midline sternotomy scars, thoracotomy scars for mitral valvotomy may be missed under the female breast).

12. Feel the apex beat – position and character.

13. Feel for left parasternal heave and thrills at the apex and on either side of the sternum.

14. Listen to the heart beginning from the apex: take care to palpate the right carotid pulse simultaneously so that the examiner notices that you are timing the various cardiac events.

    If you do not hear the mid-diastolic murmur of mitral stenosis – make sure you listen to the apex in the left lateral position with the bell of the stethoscope.

    If you hear a murmur at the apex, ensure that you get the patient to breathe in and out – the examiner will be observing whether or not you are listening for the variation in intensity with respiration.

    If you hear a pansystolic murmur, listen at the axilla (mitral regurgitant murmurs are conducted to the axilla).

15. Using the diaphragm of your stethoscope listen at the apex, below the sternum, along the left sternal edge, the second right intercostal space and the neck (for ejection systolic murmur of aortic stenosis, aortic sclerosis).

16. Request the patient to sit forward and listen with the diaphragm along the left sternal edge in the 3rd intercostal area with the patient's breath held in expiration for early diastolic murmur of aortic regurgitation.

17. Tell the examiner that you would like to do the following:

    • Listen to lung bases for signs of cardiac failure.
    • Check for sacral oedema.
    • Examine the liver (tender liver of cardiac failure), splenomegaly (endocarditis).
    • Check the blood pressure.
    • Check the peripheral pulses and also check for radiofemoral delay.

Case 1 | Mitral Stenosis

Instruction

Examine this patient's cardiovascular system.

Salient features

- Pulse is regular or irregularly irregular secondary to associated atrial fibrillation.
- Jugular venous pressure (JVP) may be raised.
- Malar flush.
- Apex beat in the left 5th intercostal space just medial to the mid-clavicular line – tapping in nature.
- Left parasternal heave.
- First heart sound is loud.
- Mid-diastolic rumbling, low pitched murmur is present – best heard in left lateral position on expiration.
- Pulmonary component of the second sound (P_2) is loud.

Note. In patients with valvular lesions the candidate would be expected to comment on rhythm, presence of heart failure and signs of pulmonary hypertension.

Questions

What is the commonest cause of mitral stenosis?

Rheumatic heart disease.

What are the complications?

- Left atrial enlargement and atrial fibrillation.
- Systemic embolisation, especially cerebral hemispheres.
- Pulmonary hypertension and right heart failure.
- Tricuspid regurgitation.

What are the signs of pulmonary hypertension?

- Large 'a' waves in the JVP.

- Left parasternal heave.
- Loud or palpable P_2.
- Ejection click in the pulmonary area.
- Early diastolic murmur (Graham Steell murmur) due to pulmonary regurgitation.

How does one clinically determine the severity of the stenosis?

- The narrower the distance between the second sound and the opening snap, the greater the severity.
- The longer the duration of the diastolic murmur, the greater the severity. Note that in tight mitral stenosis the murmur may be less prominent or inaudible and the findings may be primarily those of pulmonary hypertension.

What are the radiological features of mitral stenosis?

- Congested upper lobe veins.
- Double silhouette due to enlarged left atrium.
- Straightening of the left border of the heart due to prominent pulmonary conus and filling of the pulmonary bay by the enlarged left atrium.
- Kerley B lines (horizontal lines in the region of the costophrenic angles).

Uncommonly:

- Left bronchus may be horizontal due to an enlarged left atrium.
- Mottling due to secondary pulmonary haemosiderosis.

■ What are the indications for surgery?

- Patients with severe symptoms and significant mitral stenosis.
- Patients with pulmonary hypertension, even if minimally symptomatic.
- Recurrent thromboembolic events despite therapeutic anticoagulants.

Which surgical procedures are used to treat mitral stenosis?

- Mitral valvotomy.
- Commissurotomy.
- Valve replacement.
- Balloon valvuloplasty.

What are the indications for cardiac catheterization in such patients?

- Concomitant coronary artery disease.
- Technically difficult and nonconclusive echocardiogram.

- There is associated mitral regurgitation (in which case commissurotomy is untenable) or there are other valvular lesions, e.g. aortic insufficiency.

Mention some rarer causes of mitral stenosis.

- Calcification of mitral annulus and leaflets.
- Rheumatoid arthritis, systemic lupus erythematosus (SLE).
- Malignant carcinoid.
- Congenital stenosis.

Which conditions simulate mitral stenosis?

- Left atrial myxoma.
- Ball valve thrombus in the left atrium.
- Cor triatriatum (a rare congenital heart condition).

Have you heard of Ortner's syndrome?

It refers to the hoarseness of voice caused by left vocal cord paralysis associated with enlarged left atrium in mitral stenosis.

What are the main pathological types of rheumatic stenosis?

- Commissural type, in which there is fusion of commissures with little involvement of the chordae and/or the cusps.
- Chordae type, in which there is fusion and thickening of the chordae, resulting in shortening and diminished mobility of the leaflets.
- Leaflet type, in which the leaflets become stiff, rigid and calcified.

N Ortner (1865–1935), Professor of Medicine, Vienna, described the syndrome in 1897.
PJ Kerley (1900–1978), British Radiologist.
Paul Wood was consultant Cardiologist at the Hammersmith and National Heart Hospitals and his clinical skills are legendary. He had profound influence on British Cardiology.
Arthur Selzer, Professor of Cardiology, University of Stanford was born in Poland and he worked at the Hammersmith Hospital under the late Paul Wood. He died recently in 1992 and is best known for his contribution to quinidine syncope.

References

Bonchek, LI (1980) Indications for surgery of the mitral valve. *Am J Cardiol* **46:** 155.
Coulshed, N, Epstein, EJ, McKendrick, CS et al (1970) Systemic embolization in mitral disease. *Br Heart J* **32:** 26.
Olesen, KH (1962) The natural history of 271 patients with mitral stenosis under medical treatment. *Br Heart J* **24:** 349.
Rahimtoola, SH (1987) Catheter balloon valvuloplasty of aortic and mitral stenosis. *Circulation* **75:** 895.

Selzer, A & Cohn, KE (1972) Natural history of mitral stenosis: a review. *Circulation* **45**: 878.
Wood, P (1954) An appreciation of mitral stenosis. *Br Med J* **1**: 1051, 1113.

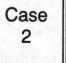 Case 2 | # Mitral Regurgitation

Instruction

Examine this patient's heart.

Salient features

- Apex beat will be displaced downwards and outwards and will be forceful in character.
- First heart sound will be soft and a third heart sound is common.
- Pansystolic murmur conducted to the axilla is heard, best detected with the diaphragm and on expiration. (**Note.** it is important to be sure that there is no associated tricuspid regurgitation.)

Questions

Mention some causes of mitral regurgitation.

- Rheumatic heart disease.
- Infective endocarditis.
- Papillary muscle dysfunction.
- Mitral valve prolapse.
- Cardiomyopathy.
- Connective tissue disorders.

How would you investigate this patient?

- Electrocardiogram (ECG) looking for left ventricular hypertrophy, atrial fibrillation.
- Chest X-ray (CXR) looking for large heart, left atrial enlargement.
- Doppler ultrasound.
- Cardiac catheterisation.

How would you differentiate between mitral regurgitation and tricuspid regurgitation?

	Mitral regurgitation	Tricuspid regurgitation
Pulse	Jerky pulse	Normal
JVP		Prominent 'v' wave
Palpation	Left ventricular heave	Left parasternal heave
Auscultation	Pansystolic murmur	Pansystolic murmur
	Intensity increases with expiration	Intensity increases with inspiration
	Radiates to the axilla	
Other signs		Hepatic pulsations

What are the causes of pansystolic murmur over the precordium?

- Mitral regurgitation.
- Tricuspid regurgitation.
- Ventricular septal defect (VSD).

■ How would you determine the severity of this lesion?

- Clinical examination shows that the larger the left ventricle the greater the severity.
- Colour Doppler quantifies the severity into three grades.

What are the indications for surgery in this patient?

- Moderate to severe symptoms despite medical therapy, provided that left ventricular function is adequate.
- Patients with minimal or no symptoms should be followed up every 6 months by echocardiographic or radionuclide assessment of left ventricular size and systolic function. When the ejection fraction falls to 55%, mitral valve repair or replacement should be considered.

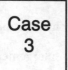

Case 3

Mixed Mitral Valve Disease

Instruction

Listen to this patient's heart.

Salient features

Patient will have signs of both mitral stenosis and regurgitation. The candidate would be expected to indicate the dominant lesion (see below).

	Dominant mitral stenosis	Dominant mitral regurgitation
Apex beat	Tapping, not displaced	Displaced
First heart sound	Loud	Soft
Third heart sound	Absent	Present

A third heart sound in mitral regurgitation indicates that any associated mitral stenosis is insignificant.

Note. There may be patients who do not have clear-cut signs such as a loud first heart sound with a displaced apex; in such cases you must say that it is difficult to ascertain clinically the dominant lesion and that cardiac catheterisation should resolve the issue.

Look carefully for mitral valvotomy scars in all patients (patients with previous valvotomy may have regurgitation and re-stenosis).

Questions

What is the cause of mitral stenosis with regurgitation?

Mixed mitral valve disease is usually due to chronic rheumatic heart disease.

What are the approximate frequencies with which various valves are affected by rheumatic heart disease?

• Mitral valve, 80%.

- Aortic valve, 50%.
- Combined mitral and aortic valve lesion, 20%.
- Tricuspid valve, 10%.
- Pulmonary valve, <1%.

Joseph K Perloff, contemporary Professor of Cardiology, Los Angeles whose chief interest is congenital heart disease.
William C Roberts, contemporary US cardiac pathologist and Editor of American Journal of Cardiology.

References

Bonchek, LI (1980) Indications for surgery of the mitral valve. *Am J Cardiol* **46**: 155.
Ellis, LB, Singh, JB, Morales, DD et al (1973) Fifteen to twenty years study of one thousand patients undergoing closed mitral valvuloplasty. *Circulation* **48**: 357.
Roberts, WC & Perloff, JK (1972) Mitral valvular disease. A clinicopathologic survey of the conditions causing the mitral valve to function abnormally. *Ann Intern Med* **77**: 939.

| Case 4 | Aortic Regurgitation |

Instruction

Examine this patient's cardiovascular system.
Examine this patient's heart.

Salient features

- The pulse may be large volume and collapsing.
- Head nodding in time with the heart beat or du Musset's sign may be present.
- Visible carotid pulsation may be obvious in the neck – dancing carotids or Corrigan's sign.

- Apex beat will be displaced outwards and forceful.
- Early diastolic murmur is heard at the left sternal edge with the diaphragm – if not apparent it is important to sit the patient forward and auscultate with the patient's breath held at the end of expiration.
- An ejection systolic murmur may be heard at the base of the heart in severe aortic regurgitation. This murmur may be loud as grade 5 or 6 and an underlying organic stenosis can be ruled out only by investigations.

- Tell the examiner you would like to do the following:
    Check the blood pressure.
    Look for signs of hyperdynamic circulation – auscultate over the femoral arteries for 'pistol shots' (Traube's sign) and a to-and-fro murmur (Duroziez's sign), and look for capillary pulsations in the nail bed (Quincke's sign).
    Check pupils for Argyll Robertson pupil of syphilis.
    Look for stigmata of Marfan's syndrome – high arched palate, arm span greater than height.
    Check joints for ankylosing spondylitis and rheumatoid arthritis.

Questions

Mention a few causes of chronic aortic regurgitation.

- Rheumatic fever
- Bacterial endocarditis.
- Syphilis.
- Hypertension.
- Seronegative arthropathy.
- Bicuspid aortic valve.

What are the clinical signs of severity?

- Wide pulse pressure.
- Soft second heart sound.
- The duration of the decrescendo diastolic murmur.
- Presence of left ventricular third heart sound.
- Austin Flint murmur.
- Signs of left ventricular failure.

Do characteristics of the early diastolic murmur correlate with severity?

Yes. In mild aortic regurgitation the murmur is short but as the severity of the regurgitation increases the murmur becomes longer and louder. In very severe regurgitation the murmur may extend throughout diastole.

What is an Austin Flint murmur?

It is an apical, low-pitched diastolic murmur due to vibration of the anterior mitral cusp.

■ Mention a few causes of acute aortic regurgitation.
● Infective endocarditis.
● Aortic dissection.
● Trauma.
● Failure of prosthetic valve.
● Rupture of aneurysm of sinus of Valsalva.

How is aortic regurgitation treated?

Aortic regurgitation is usually treated surgically. The timing of surgery is important and depends on severity of symptoms and extent of left ventricular dysfunction. Indications for surgery include:

● Symptoms of heart failure and diminished left ventricular function (an ejection fraction less than 50% but more than 20–30%).
● Patients with severe symptoms but normal left ventricular size and systolic function should be followed up at 6-monthly intervals by echocardiography or radionuclide ventriculography.

In the young, mechanical prostheses are used as the valves are more durable. Tissue valves are prone to calcification and degeneration.,
    In the elderly and in those for whom anticoagulants are contra-indicated, tissue valves are preferred.

Austin Flint (1812–1886) was one of the founders of Buffalo Medical College, New York, and reported the murmur in two patients with aortic regurgitation, confirmed by postmortem. He also held chairs at New Orleans, Chicago, Louisville and New York.
HI Quincke (1842–1922) was a German physician who described angioneurotic oedema and benign intracranial hypertension.
PI Durozicz (1826–1897), a French physician, was widely acclaimed for his articles on mitral stenosis.
L Traube (1818–1876), a German physician, was the first to describe pulsus bigeminus.
Antonio Maria Valsalva (1666–1723) was an Italian anatomist and surgeon who discovered the labyrinth and developed the Valsalva manoeuvre to remove foreign bodies from the ear.

References

Nishimura, RA, McGoon, MD, Schaff, HV & Giuliani ER (1988) Chronic aortic regurgitation. Indications for operation. *Mayo Clinic Proc* **63**: 270.

Siemienczuk, D, Greenberg, B, Morris, C et al (1989) Chronic aortic insufficiency. Factors associated with progression to aortic valve replacement. *Ann Intern Med* **110:** 587.

Case 5	Aortic Stenosis

Instruction

Examine this patient's heart.

Salient features

- Low volume or anacrotic pulse.
- Apex beat is heaving in nature but is not displaced. (A displaced apex beat indicates left ventricular dilatation and severe disease.)
- Systolic thrill over the aortic area and carotids.
- Ejection systolic murmur at the base of the heart conducted to the carotids.

Note. Valvular stenosis may be accompanied by an ejection click; aortic component of second sound will be soft, and in severe stenosis there may be a reversal of the split second sound. (Listen carefully for an early diastolic murmur as mild aortic regurgitation often accompanies aortic stenosis.)

- Tell the examiner you would like to check the blood pressure, keeping in mind that the pulse pressure is low in moderate to severe stenosis.

Questions

How would you differentiate aortic stenosis from aortic sclerosis?

Aortic sclerosis is seen in the elderly; the pulse is normal volume, the apex beat is not shifted and the murmur is localised.

Mention some causes of aortic stenosis.

- Under the age of 60: rheumatic, congenital.
- Between 60 and 75 years: calcified bicuspid aortic valve, especially in men.
- Over the age of 75: degenerative calcification.

Mention other causes of ejection systolic murmur at the base of the heart.

- Pulmonary stenosis.
- Hypertrophic obstructive cardiomyopathy.
- Supravalvular aortic stenosis.

How may this patient present?

With one of the following:

- Angina.
- Dyspnoea.
- Syncope.
- Sudden death.

What investigations would you do?

- ECG looking for left ventricular hypertrophy, ST–T changes.
- CXR looking for poststenotic dilatation of aorta and valve calcification.
- Echocardiogram.
- Cardiac catheterisation, looking at coronary arteries, mitral and aortic valves.

What are the complications of aortic stenosis?

- Left ventricular failure.
- Infective endocarditis (in 10% of cases).

What are the clinical signs of severity of aortic stenosis?

- Narrow pulse pressure.
- Soft second sound.
- Narrow or reverse split second sound.
- Systolic thrill and heaving apex beat.
- Fourth heart sound.
- Cardiac failure.

■ How would you manage this patient?

- If the patient is asymptomatic and valvular gradient is less than 50 mmHg then observe the patient.

- Valve replacement in the following circumstances:
  The patient is symptomatic or the valvular gradient is more than 60 mmHg.
  The valve area is less than $0.7\,cm^2$ (normal area $3-4\,cm^2$).
- Often, patients require coronary artery bypass grafts during aortic valve replacement.
- Balloon valvuloplasty is a new therapeutic option instead of valve replacement.

If this patient had bleeding per rectum what unusual cause would come to mind?

Angiodysplasia of the colon.

If this patient was icteric and had haemolytic anaemia what would the mechanism be?

Microangiopathic haemolysis has been described in severe aortic stenosis manifesting with anaemia and icterus.

Williams syndrome is characterised by elfin facies, supravalvular aortic stenosis and hypercalcaemia.
JCP Williams, New Zealand physician.

References

Galloway, SJ, Casarella, WJ & Shimkin PM (1974) Vascular malformations of the right colon as a cause of bleeding in patients with aortic stenosis. *Radiology* **113:** 11.

Lombard, JT & Selzer, A (1987) Valvular aortic stenosis: a clinical and hemodynamic profile of patients. *Ann Intern Med* **106:** 292.

Marsh, GW & Lewis, SM (1969) Cardiac hemolytic anemia. *Semin Hematol* **6:** 133.

Safian, RD, Berman, AD, Diver, DJ et al (1988) Balloon aortic valvuloplasty in 170 consecutive patients. *N Engl J Med* **319:** 125.

Selzer, A (1987) Changing aspects of the natural history of valvular aortic stenosis. *N Engl J Med* **317:** 91.

Wood, P (1958) Aortic stenosis. *Am J Cardiol* **1:** 533.

Case 6 | Mixed Aortic Valve Lesion

Instruction

Examine this patient's heart.
Examine this patient's cardiovascular system.
Examine this patient's pulse.

Salient features

- Pulse may be bisferious, small volume or large volume depending on the dominant lesion.
- Displaced apex beat.
- Early diastolic murmur of aortic regurgitation.
- Ejection systolic murmur of aortic stenosis.

- Tell the examiner that you would like to check the blood pressure, in particular to determine the pulse pressure (systolic minus the diastolic pressure).
- In *dominant aortic stenosis*:
  Pulse volume is small.
  Blood pressure is normal and pulse pressure is narrow.
- In *dominant aortic regurgitation*:
  Pulse is collapsing.
  Pulse pressure is wide.

Questions

What are the common causes of mixed aortic lesions?

- Rheumatic heart disease.
- Bicuspid aortic valve.

Case 7	Mixed Mitral and Aortic Valve Disease

Instruction

Examine this patient's cardiovascular system.
Examine this patient's heart.
Examine this patient's precordium.

Salient features

- Pulse may be small volume (either due to dominant aortic stenosis or mitral stenosis), regular or irregularly irregular.
- Apex beat may be displaced.
- Left parasternal heave.
- Mid-diastolic murmur of mitral stenosis.
- Pansystolic murmur of mitral regurgitation.
- Ejection systolic murmur of aortic stenosis at the base of the heart.
- Early diastolic murmur of aortic regurgitation heard with the patient sitting forward on end expiration.

Note. If the apex beat is not displaced in such mixed lesions then mitral stenosis is the dominant lesion. (However, if the mitral stenosis developed earlier it can mask the signs of a significant aortic stenosis.)

Questions

Mention a few causes of combined aortic and mitral valve disease.

- Rheumatic valvular disease.
- Infective endocarditis.
- Collagen degenerative disorder, e.g. Marfan's syndrome.
- Calcific changes in the aortic and mitral valve apparatus.

■ What are the indications for surgery?

- New York Heart Association (NYHA) class III status.
- Class II status where there is volume overload of the left ventricle, e.g. in severe aortic regurgitation with moderate mitral valve disease or severe mitral regurgitation with moderate aortic stenosis and regurgitation.

Note. The NYHA grading of cardiac status is as follows:
Grade I, uncompromised.
Grade II, slightly compromised.
Grade III, moderately compromised.
Grade IV, severely compromised.

Robert Frye, contemporary Professor and Chairman of the Dept of Medicine, Mayo Clinic whose chief interest is cardiovascular diseases.

References

Stephenson, LW, Harken, AH et al (1984) Combined aortic and mitral valve replacement: changes in practice and prognosis. *Circulation* **69:** 640.
Terazi, AK, Cokkinos, DV, Leachman, RD et al (1970) Combined mitral and aortic valve disease. *Am J Cardiol* **25:** 588.

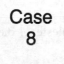

Case 8   Hypertension

Instruction

This patient has hypertension; would you like to examine him (her)?

Salient features

- Comment on Cushingoid facies if present.
- Look for radiofemoral delay of coarctation of aorta.
- Palpate the apex for left ventricular hypertrophy.
- Look for signs of cardiac failure.
- Examine the fundus for changes of hypertensive retinopathy.
- Listen for renal artery bruit of renal artery stenosis.

- Tell the examiner that you would like to check urine for protein (renal failure) and sugar (associated diabetes).

Questions

How would you investigate a patient with hypertension in out-patients?

- Full blood count (FBC).
- Urine for sugar, albumin and specific gravity.
- Urea, electrolytes and serum creatinine.
- Fasting lipids, serum uric acid.
- ECG.
- CXR.

What are the causes of hypertension?

- Unknown.
- Renal: glomerulonephritis, diabetic nephropathy, renal artery stenosis, pyelonephritis.
- Endocrine: Cushing's syndrome, steroid therapy, phaeochromocytoma.
- Others: coarctation of aorta, contraceptives, toxaemia of pregnancy.

How would you manage a patient with mild hypertension?

- General measures:
  Diet: weight reduction in obese patients, low-cholesterol diets for associated hyperlipidaemia, salt restriction.
  Stop smoking.
  Reduce heavy alcohol consumption.
- Drug treatment:
  Beta blockers in nonsmoking males.
  Bendrofluazide in women and male smokers.

What special investigations would you do to screen for an underlying cause.

- Renal digital subtraction angiogram.
- 24-hour urinary cathecholamines – at least three samples (phaeochromocytoma).
- Overnight dexamethasone suppression test.

Sir SW Peart, Emeritus Professor of Medicine at St Mary's Hospital Medical School, London, purified and sequenced angiotensin II and was involved in pioneering work in the field of hypertension.

References

Swales, JD (1991) First line treatment in hypertension. *Br Med J* **301:** 1172.

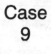 **Atrial Fibrillation**

Case
9

Instruction

Examine this patient's pulse.

Salient features

- Irregularly irregular pulse (patients are often digitalised and in slow atrial fibrillation).

- Ask the examiner if you may perform the following checks:
    Examine the heart for mitral valvular lesion.
    Check the blood pressure for hypertension.
    Ask the patient for history of ischaemic heart disease.
    Check the patient's thyroid status for thyrotoxicosis.

Questions

What are the common causes of atrial fibrillation?

- Mitral valvular disease in the young and middle aged.
- Ischaemic heart disease or hypertension in the elderly.
- Thyrotoxicosis (atrial fibrillation may be the only clinical feature in the elderly).
- Constrictive pericarditis.

Mention common sites of systemic embolisation.

Brain, leg, kidney, superior mesenteric artery, coronary artery and spleen.

At the bedside how would you differentiate atrial fibrillation from multiple ventricular ectopics?

If the patient is not in heart failure, exercise the patient: after exercise, ventricular ectopics tend to diminish in frequency whereas there is no change in the rhythm of atrial fibrillation.

■ Mention a few causes of irregularly irregular pulse.

Atrial fibrillation, atrial flutter with varying block, multiple ventricular ectopics.

In which congenital disorders is atrial fibrillation common?

Atrial septal defect (ASD), Ebstein's anomaly.

What do you understand by the term 'lone atrial fibrillation'?

Lone atrial fibrillation occurs in the absence of cardiopulmonary disease or a history of hypertension and before the age of 60. Such patients are associated with a very low risk of stroke (0.5% per year).

How would you treat a patient with atrial fibrillation?

- Attempt to slow ventricular rate using digoxin, propranolol, verapamil or amiodarone.
- Attempt to restore sinus rhythm by cardioversion if the following conditions apply:
    Left atrial size by echocardiogram is less than 4.5 cm (a left atrial size greater than 4.5 cm is not associated with long-term maintenance of sinus rhythm).
- Duration of the arrhythmia of acute atrial fibrillation is likely to remain in sinus rhythm.
- Anticoagulation with warfarin is advised for certain patients:
    Undergoing cardioversion (electrical or drug).
    Underlying mitral valve disease.
    In left ventricular failure.
    Cardiomyopathy.
    Above 60 years of age.

Mention a few drugs used to restore sinus rhythm.

Procainamide, disopyramide or quinidine for 2–3 days restores sinus rhythm in up to 30% of patients.

W Ebstein (1836–1912), a German physician, wrote articles on renal disease, pericardial effusion and diabetes.

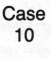

Case 10   Palpitations

Instruction

This man has palpitations; would you like to ask him a few questions?

Salient features

Ask the following questions:

- Are the palpitations regular or irregular?
- Is the onset abrupt (paroxysmal tachyarrhythmias)?
- How frequent are the palpitations?
- What is the duration of each episode?
- Is each episode followed by polyuria (seen in supraventricular tachycardia)?
- Is there any relation to exercise?
- What happens on standing (postural hypotension)?
- Are there any precipitating factors such as coffee, tea, alcohol, or medications such as thyroid extract, ephedrine, aminophylline, monoamine oxidase inhibitors?
- Are there any associated symptoms such as chest pain, shortness of breath?

Questions

What are the causes?

- Extrasystoles.
- Tachycardias or bradycardias.

- Drugs (see above).
- Others: thyrotoxicosis, hypoglycaemia, unaccustomed exertion, phaeochromocytoma, fever.
- Anxiety state (also known as Da Costa's syndrome or cardiac neurosis).

How would you investigate a patient suspected to have a disorder of cardiac rhythm?

- 12-lead ECG (look for evidence of a rhythm disturbance and pre-excitation syndrome).
- Continuous ambulatory (Holter) electrocardiography.

John Camm, Regius Professor of Medicine and Cardiology, St George's Hospital, London, whose chief interest is cardiac arrhythmias.
JM Da Costa (1833–1900), Professor of Medicine at the Jefferson Medical College, Philadelphia.

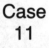

Case 11 | Slow Pulse Rate

Instruction

Examine this patient's pulse.

Salient features

- Pulse rate of less than 60 beats per minute.
- Pulse may be either regular or irregular.
- If the pulse is irregular tell the examiner that you would like to do the following:

    Get the patient to stand and then count his or her pulse rate (in complete heart block there is no increase in rate).
    Look at the JVP for cannon 'a' waves.
    Auscultate the heart for cannon first heart sound.

- Tell the examiner that you would like to take a drug history – beta blockers, digoxin, verapamil.

Questions

What are the causes of sinus bradycardia?

- Physical fitness in athletes.
- Acute myocardial infarction.
- Drugs (beta blockers, digitalis).
- Myxoedema.
- Obstructive jaundice.
- Increased intracranial pressure.
- Hypothermia.
- Hyperkalaemia.

■ What are the indications of temporary cardiac pacing in brady-arrhythmias?

- Symptomatic second or third degree heart block due to transient drug intoxication or electrolyte imbalance.
- Complete heart block, Mobitz II or bifasicular block in the setting of acute myocardial infarct.
- Symptomatic sinus bradycardia, atrial fibrillation with a slow ventricular response.

What are the indications for permanent pacing in bradyarrhythmias?

- Symptomatic congenital heart block.
- Symptomatic sinus bradycardia.
- Symptomatic second or third degree heart block.

Which drug would you use to treat bradycardia seen in the setting of an acute myocardial infarction?

Intravenous atropine 0.6 mg, slowly (up to 3 mg in 24 hours).

Have you heard of Stokes–Adams syndrome?

It refers to syncope or fits occurring during complete heart block.

W Stokes (1804–1878), Regius Professor of Medicine in Dublin, graduated from Edinburgh. R Adams (1791–1875), Professor of Surgery in Dublin, was an authority on gout and arthritis.

Case 12	Gallop Rhythm

Instruction

Listen to the precordium.
Examine this patient's heart.

Salient features

- Presence of an abnormal third or fourth heart sound with tachycardia (the presence of a normal third or fourth heart sound does not connote a gallop rhythm unless there is associated tachycardia).
- Auscultate with the bell as both third and fourth heart sounds are low pitched.
- Gallop rhythm due to third heart sound seems to sound like 'Kentucky' whereas that due to the fourth heart sound seems to sound like 'Tennessee'.

Note. A left ventricular third heart sound is best heard at the apex whereas the right ventricular third heart sound is best heard along the left sternal border.

Questions

What is the expression used when both the third and fourth heart sounds are heard with tachycardia?

This is known as a summation gallop.

What is the mechanism of production of the third heart sound?

It is due to rapid ventricular filling in early diastole.

What is the mechanism of production of the fourth heart sound?

It is due to vigorous contraction of the atria (atrial systole) and is hence heard towards the end of diastole.

■ What are the causes of a third heart sound?

- Physiological: in normal children and young adults.

- Pathological:
    Heart failure.
    Mitral regurgitation.

What are the causes of a fourth heart sound?

- Normal: in the elderly.
- Pathological:
    Acute myocardial infarction.
    Aortic stenosis.
    Hypertension.

Peter Sever, contemporary Professor of Clinical Pharmacology, St Mary's Hospital, London, whose chief interests include hypertension and cardiovascular prevention.

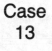

Case 13 | Myocardial Infarction

Instruction

This patient has had a myocardial infarction; would you like to examine him (her)?

Salient features

- Hands: nicotine staining of fingers.
- Pulse: check pulse rate and rhythm.
- JVP may be raised in cardiac failure or right ventricular infarction.
- Eyes: look for arcus senilis, xanthelasma.
- Cardiac apex: look for double apical impulse.
- Auscultate for fourth heart sound, pericardial rub, pansystolic murmur of papillary muscle dysfunction.
- Tell the examiner that you would like to examine the following:
    The chest for crackles.

The abdomen for tender liver of cardiac failure.
The legs for deep vein thrombosis.

Questions

How would you manage a patient with an uncomplicated myocardial infarction in a coronary care unit?

- Bed rest.
- Oxygen.
- Pain relief.
- Sedation.
- Aspirin 150 mg Stat.
- Intravenous streptokinase if no contraindications.

What are the complications of myocardial infarction?

- Rhythm disorders: tachycardia, bradycardia, ventricular ectopics, ventricular fibrillation, atrial fibrillation, atrial tachycardia.
- Heart failure: acute pulmonary oedema.
- Circulatory failure: cardiogenic shock.
- Infarction of the papillary muscle: mitral regurgitation and acute pulmonary oedema.
- Rupture of the ventricle, leading to cardiac tamponade.
- Rupture of the interventricular septum.
- Thromboembolism – cerebral or peripheral.
- Venous thrombosis.
- Pericarditis.
- Dressler's syndrome – characterised by persistent pyrexia, pericarditis, pleurisy.

■ What is a silent myocardial infarct?

A painless infarct, common in diabetics and the elderly; it may present with the complications of myocardial infarction.

What are the contraindications for streptokinase therapy?

- History of recent bleeding.
- Stroke.
- Severe hypertension.
- Recent surgery or any other invasive procedure within the previous 10 days.
- Proliferative diabetic retinopathy.
- If the patient has received streptokinase in the previous 6 months.
- Concurrent use of anticoagulants.
- Concurrent terminal illness.

Peter Sleight, contemporary Professor of Cardiology at Oxford, is the chairman of the multicentric ISIS trials.
W Dressler (1890–1969), US physician educated in Vienna.
L David Hillis, contemporary Professor of Cardiology, University of Texas, Dallas; his chief interest is coronary artery disease.

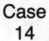

Case 14 | Jugular Venous Pulse

Instruction

Examine this patient's neck.
Examine this patient's cardiovascular system.

Salient features

- The JVP is raised . . . cm above the angle of Louis (manubriosternal angle). Remember that the JVP may be raised to the level of the ear lobes.
- Comment on the wave form (timing it with the carotid pulse):
  'v' waves of tricuspid regurgitation.
  Cannon waves of heart block.
  Absent 'a' waves in atrial fibrillation (irregular carotid pulse).
  Large 'a' waves of pulmonary hypertension, pulmonary stenosis, tricuspid stenosis.

- Tell the examiner that you would like to look for other signs of heart failure:
  Basal crackles.
  Dependent oedema (ankle and sacral oedema).
  Tender hepatomegaly.

Questions

What other signs of tricuspid regurgitation do you know?

- Pansystolic murmur at the left lower sternal border which increases in intensity on inspiration (Carvallo's sign).
- Pulsatile liver.

What do you know about the wave forms in the jugular pulse?

- The 'a' wave is due to atrial contraction and is presystolic.
- The 'c' wave is due to closure of the tricuspid valve.
- The 'v' wave is due to venous return to the right heart (*not* due to ventricular contraction).
- The 'x' descent is due to atrial relaxation.
- The 'y' descent is produced by opening of tricuspid valve and rapid inflow of blood into the right ventricle.

What are causes of a raised JVP?

- Congestive cardiac failure.
- Cor pulmonale.
- Tricuspid stenosis or tricuspid regurgitation.
- Pulmonary hypertension.
- Complete heart block.
- Nonpulsatile neck veins are seen in superior vena caval obstruction.

■ What is Kussmaul's sign?

Normally there is an inspiratory decrease in JVP. In constrictive pericarditis there is an inspiratory increase in JVP. It is also seen in severe right heart failure regardless of aetiology. It is caused by the inability of the heart to accept the increase in right ventricular volume without a marked increase in the filling pressure.

Adolf Kussmaul (1822–1902) was a Professor of Medicine successively at Heidelberg, Enlargen, Freiburg and Strasbourg and coined the term 'polyarteritis nodosa'. Kussmaul breathing is a deep sighing respiration seen when the arterial pH is low.
Thomas W Smith, Professor of Cardiology at Harvard Medical School; his interests include digitalis glycosides and molecular mechanisms of cardiac contractility.
Phillip Poole-Wilson, contemporary Professor of Cardiology at the Royal Brompton and National Heart and Lung Institutes, London; his chief interest is cardiac failure.

References

Kussmaul, A (1873) Uber Schwielige Mediastino-pericarditis und Den Paradoxen Pulse. *Berl Klin Wochenschr* **10**: 433.

Case 15 | Infective Endocarditis

Instruction

This patient is suspected to have endocarditis; would you like to examine him (her)?

Salient features

Look for the following signs:

- Anaemia.
- Clubbing.
- Splinter haemorrhages in the nails.
- Osler's nodes (see below).
- Janeway lesions (see below).
- Petechiae – conjunctival and skin.

- Listen to the heart for murmurs and look for signs of cardiac failure.
- Tell the examiner that you would like to do the following:
    Examine the fundus for Roth's spots.
    Examine the abdomen for splenomegaly.
    Test the urine for microscopic haematuria.
    Take a history of recent dental procedure.
    Remember that ostium secundum atrial septal defects almost never have infective endocarditis.

Questions

What do you know about Libman–Sacks endocarditis?

It is a noninfective endocarditis seen in SLE and is largely a pathological finding.

How would you investigate such a patient?

- Test the urine for microscopic haematuria.
- Measure FBC to show normocytic, normochromic anaemia and raised white cell count.
- Test for raised erythrocyte sedimentation rate (ESR).

- Blood culture: take three samples from different sites in 24 hours.
- Echocardiogram may show vegetations. A negative study does not rule out endocarditis as vegetations less than 3–4 mm in size cannot be detected. Furthermore, all the leaflets of the aortic, tricuspid and pulmonary valves may not be visualised in every patient.

What are the major manifestations of bacterial endocarditis?

- Manifestations of a systemic infection: fever, weight loss, pallor, splenomegaly.
- Manifestations of intravascular phenomenon: cardiac failure, changing murmurs, petechiae, Roth's spots, Osler's nodes, Janeway lesions, splinter haemorrhages, stroke, infarction of viscera, mycotic aneurysm.
- Manifestations of immunological reactions: arthralgia, finger clubbing, uraemia.

How would you treat a patient suspected to have endocarditis?

Until the bacteriology results are available, with intravenous Benzyl-penicillin and Gentamicin. In severely ill patients intravenous Cloxa-cillin would be added to this regime.

Name the common organisms found in infective endocarditis.

Streptococcus viridans, Staphylococcus aureus, Strep. faecalis, fungi.

What precaution would you take to prevent bacterial endocarditis?

Antibiotic prophylaxis before any dental, gastrointestinal, urological or gynaecological procedure.

What are Osler's nodes?

Tender, erythematous, pea-sized nodules seen in the pulp of the fingers. They are caused by inflammation around the site of infected emboli lodged in distal arterioles.

What are Janeway lesions?

Flat, nontender red spots found on the palms and soles, and they blanch on pressure.

■ Mention a few poor prognostic factors.

- Heart failure.
- Nonstreptococcal endocarditis, especially *Staph. aureus*, fungal endocarditis.
- Infection of prosthetic valve.

- Elderly patients.
- Valve ring or myocardial abscess.

Mention a few conditions which can simulate clinical manifestations of infective endocarditis.

- Atrial myxoma.
- Nonbacterial endocarditis.
- SLE.
- Sickle cell disease.

What are splinter haemorrhages caused by?

The probable cause is embolisation to linear capillaries in the nail bed.

What are the indications for surgery?

- Positive blood cultures or relapse after several days of best available antibiotic therapy requires valve replacement.
- Drainage of myocardial or valve ring abscesses.
- Patients with aortic valve endocarditis who develop second or third degree heart block.
- Prosthetic valve replacement for nonstreptococcal endocarditis, valve dysfunction, valve dehiscence or myocardial invasion.

What do you understand by the term 'marantic endocarditis'?

- Marantic or Libman–Sacks endocarditis is seen in SLE and is an autopsy diagnosis. It is rarely clinically significant.

Sir William Osler (1849–1919) was successively a Professor of Medicine at Montreal, Pennsylvania, Baltimore and Oxford. He was reputed to be a brilliant clinician and educationist.
M Roth (1839–1914), Professor of Pathology at Basel, Switzerland.
EG Janeway (1841–1911) followed Austin Flint as Professor of Medicine at Bellevue Hospital, New York.
E Libman (1872–1946), US physician.
B Sacks (1873–1939), US physician who also wrote on Hindu medicine.
Celia Oakely is Professor of Cardiology at the Hammersmith Hospital, London.

Case 16	Prosthetic Heart Valves

Instruction

Listen to this patient's heart.

Salient features

- *Mitral* valve prostheses can be recognised by their site, metallic first heart sound, a normal second sound and a metallic opening snap.
- Systolic flow murmurs are often also present and it is important to note that this does *not* indicate that there is valve malfunction. Diastolic flow murmurs may be heard normally over disc valves.

- *Aortic* valve prostheses may be recognised by their site, a normal first heart sound and metallic second heart sound.

- Both *mitral and aortic* valves may be replaced and both the first and second heart sounds will be metallic. The presence of a systolic murmur does not indicate valve dysfunction. However, the presence of an early diastolic murmur indicates a malfunctioning aortic valve.

Note. Comment on the midsternal, vertical thoracotomy scar, and state whether or not the metallic valve sounds are audible to the unaided ear (they are most often audible). Porcine and cadaveric heterografts do not cause metallic clicking or plopping sounds.

Questions

What are complications of prosthetic valves?

- Thromboembolism.
- Valve dysfunction, including valve leakage, valve dehiscence, and valve obstruction due to thrombosis and clogging.
- Bleeding (such as upper gastrointestinal haemorrhage) due to anticoagulants.
- Haemolysis at valve causing anaemia.

What are the causes of anaemia in such a patient?

- Bleeding due to anticoagulants.

- Haemolytic anaemia.
- Secondary to bacterial endocarditis.

What are the advantages of a porcine valve?

There is no need for chronic anticoagulation and hence it is safe in women of childbearing age and in the elderly.

■ What are the complications of a porcine heart valve?

- Degeneration with time.
- Calcification.

What are the indications of valve replacement?

- Mitral stenosis:
  Shortness of breath
  Recurrent thromboembolism despite adequate anticoagulation.
- Mitral regurgitation:
  Disabling symptoms despite medical therapy, provided that left ventricular function is adequate.
  In those who are symptomatic or with minimal symptoms, valve replacement should be considered when the ejection fraction approaches 50–55%.
- Aortic regurgitation:
  Patients with severe aortic regurgitation, symptoms of heart failure and depressed left ventricular function (unless left ventricular dysfunction is marked, i.e. ejection fraction is less than 30%). Patients with severe aortic regurgitation and normal left ventricular size and systolic function are followed up at 6-monthly intervals until deterioration is noted and then onwards more frequently.
  Patients with mild to moderate aortic regurgitation should be followed with serial, noninvasive evaluation of left ventricular end-systolic volume and function.
- Aortic stenosis:
  Symptomatic patients.
  Asymptomatic patients with valve areas less than $0.8 \, cm^2$.

What are the different kinds of mechanical valves?

The Starr–Edwards is a caged ball device and because the blood flows around the ball there is high incidence of haemolysis. The Bjork–Shiley pivoted disc valve has central flow and hence a lower incidence of haemolysis.

What kind of valve would you use to replace the mitral valve?

Mechanical prosthesis. However, patients in whom the risk posed by anticoagulants is unacceptably high may receive a bioprosthesis, but at the increased risk of a further operation at a later date.

What kind of valve would you use to replace the aortic valve?

Mechanical valves in young patients in whom the risk of porcine valve failure is higher and for whom durability of the valve is of paramount importance. Porcine valves may be considered for elderly patients whose life expectancy may not exceed that of the prosthesis used.

Note. The first aortic valve replacement (caged ball device) was performed by Dr Dwight Harken in March 1960 at Peter Brent Brigham Hospital in Boston. Shortly thereafter, Dr Nina Braunwald, at the National Institutes for Health (NIH), USA, performed a total mitral valve replacement with an artificial flexible leaflet valve.
A Starr and ML Edwards, both US physicians.

References

Bloomfield, P, Wheatley, DJ, Prescott, RJ & Miller, HC (1991) 12 year comparison of Bjork–Shiley mechanical heart valve with porcine bioprosthesis. *N Engl J Med* **324:** 573–579. (This study concludes that survival with an intact valve is better among patients with the Bjork–Shiley spherical tilting disc valve than among patients with porcine valves, but the use of the former carries an increased risk of bleeding due to anticoagulants.)

| Case 17 | Tricuspid Regurgitation |

Instruction

Examine this patient's heart.
Examine this patient's cardiovascular system.

Salient features

- Large 'v' waves in the jugular venous pulse.
- Left parasternal heave.
- Palpable or loud P_2.
- Pansystolic murmur at the left lower sternal border which increases in inspiration – Carvallo's sign.
- Right ventricular third heart sound may be present.
- Atrial fibrillation may be present.
- Listen carefully for mid-diastolic murmur of mitral stenosis.
- Look for systolic pulsations of an enlarged liver.

Questions

What are causes of tricuspid regurgitation?

- Functional:
     pulmonary hypertension;
     congestive cardiac failure.
- Rheumatic (associated with mitral and/or aortic valve disease).
- Right heart endocarditis as in drug addicts.
- Uncommon causes: carcinoid syndrome, Ebstein's anomaly, endo-myocardial fibrosis, infarction of right ventricular papillary muscles, tricuspid valve prolapse, blunt trauma to the heart.

How would you treat functional regurgitation?

Treatment of underlying cardiac failure or pulmonary hypertension.

How would you treat organic tricuspid regurgitation?

Surgically:
     Valve plication or annuloplasty.
     Valve replacement.

JMR Carvallo, Mexican cardiologist who worked in Mexico City.
RL Popp, Contemporary Professor, Stanford Medical School, USA, whose chief interest is echocardiography.

References

McMichael, J & Shillingford, JP (1957) The role of valvular incompetence in heart failure. *Br Med J* **1**: 537.
Rivero-Carvallo, JM (1946) Signo para el diagnostico de las insuficiencias tricuspideas. *Arch Inst Cardiol Mex* **16**: 531.
York, PG & Popp, RL (1984) Noninvasive estimation of right ventricular systolic pressure by Doppler ultrasound in patients with tricuspid regurgitation. *Circulation* **70**: 657.

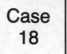

| Case 18 | Mitral Valve Prolapse |

Instruction

Examine this patient's heart.

Salient features

- Midsystolic click followed by late or midsystolic murmur.

Note. Squatting will bring the click closer to second sound and decrease the duration of the murmur. A Valsalva manoeuvre and standing have the opposite effect.

- Tell the examiner you would like to look for features of Marfan's syndrome (high arched palate, arm span greater than height).

Questions

What are the eponyms for mitral valve prolapse (MVP)?

Barlow's syndrome, click-murmur syndrome, floppy mitral valve.

What is the prevalence in the normal population?

The exact prevalence is not known but is between 2% and 10% of the population. It is present in about 7% of the females aged between 14 and 30 years.

■ What are the echocardiographic features of MVP?

- M-mode: abrupt posterior displacement of the posterior or sometimes both valve leaflets in mid- or late systole.
- 2-D: systolic displacement of one or both mitral valve leaflets into the left atrium.

What are the complications of MVP?

- Severe mitral regurgitation.
- Arrhythmias – ventricular premature contractions, ventricular tachycardia, paroxysmal supraventricular and ventricular tachycardia.
- Atypical chest pain.

- Transient ischaemic attacks (TIAs), embolism.
- Infective endocarditis in those with mitral regurgitation.
- Sudden death.

Mention a few associated conditions.

- Marfan's syndrome.
- Chronic rheumatic heart disease.
- Ischaemic heart disease.
- Cardiomyopathies.
- 20% of patients with ASD – secundum type.
- Ehlers–Danlos syndrome.
- Psoriatic arthritis.
- Ebstein's anomaly.
- SLE.

How would you manage such patients?

- Reassure the asymptomatic patient.
- Advise prophylaxis for infective endocarditis in those with the murmur.
- Relief of atypical chest pain with analgesics or beta blockers (empiric treatment).
- Aspirin or anticoagulants in those with TIAs.
- Antiarrhythmics in those with frequent tachyarrhythmias or ventricular premature contractions.

John Barlow, South African Professor of Cardiology; as a medical student he was called a 'canary' because of his penchant for rare syndromes.

References

Barlow, JB, Bosman, CK & Pocock, WA (1968) Late systolic murmurs and non ejection (mid–late) systolic clicks: an analysis of 90 patients. *Br Heart J* **30**: 203.
Devereaux, RB, Perloff, JK, Reichek, N et al (1976) Mitral valve prolapse. *Circulation* **54**: 3.
MacMahon, SW, Devereux, RB & Schron, E (guest editors) (1987) Proceedings of a National Heart, Lung and Blood Institute symposium: clinical and epidemiological issues in mitral valve prolapse. *Am Heart J* **113**: 1265 (entire issue).
Oakley, C (1985) Mitral valve prolapse. *Q J Med* **219**: 317.
Perloff, JK, Child, JS & Edwards, JE (1986) New guidelines for the clinical diagnosis of mitral valve prolapse. *Am J Cardiol* **57**: 1124.
Procacci, PN, Savran, SV, Schreiter, SL et al (1976) Prevalence of clinical mitral valve prolapse in 1169 young women. *N Engl J Med* **294**: 1986.

| Case 19 | Ventricular Septal Defect |

Instruction

Listen to this patient's heart.

Salient features

- Normal pulse.
- Normal findings on palpation (there may be either left or right ventricular enlargement).
- Loud pansystolic murmur at the left lower sternal area.

Listen for the following:

- Mid-diastolic flow murmur at the apex.
- Loud P_2 of pulmonary hypertension.
- Signs of cardiac failure.

Note. VSD is a feature of Down's syndrome.

Questions

Is the loudness of the murmur related to the size of the VSD?

No; in fact, very small defects (maladie de Roger) cause loud murmurs.

What are the causes of a VSD?

- Congenital.
- Rupture of the interventricular septum as a complication of myocardial infarction.

Where is the defect usually situated?

In the membranous portion of the interventricular septum.

Can such defects close spontaneously?

Spontaneous closure usually occurs in a small defect and occurs in early childhood in most patients.

What are the complications of a VSD?

- Congestive cardiac failure.
- Right ventricular outflow tract obstruction.
- Aortic regurgitation.
- Infective endocarditis.
- Reversal of shunt (Eisenmenger complex).

■ What types of VSD do you know?

- The supracristal type (above the crista supraventricularis).
- The infracristal defect which may be in either
  (i) the upper membranous portion, or
  (ii) the lower muscular part (less than 5% of the defects) of the inter-ventricular septum.
  Small defects (maladie de Roger).
  Swiss cheese appearance (multiple small defects).
  Large defects.
  Gerbode defect (defect opening into the right atrium).

Note. The crista supraventricularis is a muscular ridge that separates the main portion of the right ventricular cavity from the infundibular or outflow portion.

Which patients merit surgical attention?

Usually in an adult the VSD is small enough to be safely ignored, or the patient has Eisenmenger syndrome. However, there are three exceptions to this and these may benefit from surgery:
   Recurrent endocarditis.
   Development of aortic regurgitation due to prolapse of the right coronary cusp through the septal defect.
   Progressive left ventricular dilatation due to volume overload imposed by the shunt (pulmonary to systemic ratio is 3:1).

Note. If the VSD is large enough to cause heart failure or pulmonary hypertension it usually manifests in the first few years of life.

Henri Roger (1809–1891), French paediatrician, described the maladie de Roger in 1879.

References

Gerbode, F, Hultgren, H, Melrose, D & Osborn, J (1958) Syndrome of left ventricular–right atrial shunt. Successful surgical repair of defect in 5 cases, with observation of bradycardia on closure. *Ann Surg* 148: 433.

Weidman, WH, Blount, SG, DuShane, JW et al (1977) Clinical course in ventricular septal defect. *Circulation* 56(suppl 1): I–56.

Case 20	Atrial Septal Defect

Instruction

Examine this patient's heart.
Listen to his/her heart.

Salient features

- Diffuse apical impulse.
- Left parasternal heave.
- Ejection systolic murmur in the left second and third intercostal space.
- Wide, fixed split second heart sound.
- Infrequently, a mid-diastolic murmur may be heard in the tricuspid area.

- Look for signs of pulmonary hypertension (Eisenmenger syndrome).
- Examine the hands for congenital defects of the digits (Holt–Oram syndrome).

Questions

What are the types of ASD?

- Ostium secundum defect accounts for 70% of cases. The defect is in the middle portion of the atrial septum and is usually 2–4 cm in diameter (incomplete right bundle branch block pattern, QRS axis rightward).

- Sinus venosus type is a defect in the septum just below the entrance of the superior vena cava into the right atrium (leftward P wave axis so that P waves are inverted in at least one inferior lead).
- Ostium primum type is a defect in the lower part of the septum and clefts may occur in the mitral and tricuspid valves (QRS axis leftward).

What is Holt–Oram syndrome?

There is an ostium secundum ASD with a hypoplastic thumb and an accessory phalanx. In addition, the thumb lies in the same plane as the other digits. The inheritance is autosomal dominant.

At what age does reversal of shunt occur?

Usually after the end of the second decade.

What is the mechanism of fixed split second sound?

In normal individuals on inspiration there is a widening of the split between the two components of the second sound due to a delay in closure of the pulmonary valve. In ASD the effect of respiration is eliminated due to the communication between the left and right sides of the heart.

What is Lutembacher syndrome?

ASD with an acquired rheumatic mitral stenosis.

What is Fallot's trilogy?

ASD, pulmonary stenosis and right ventricular enlargement.

What are the CXR findings?

- Small aortic knob.
- Large pulmonary conus.
- Very large hilar arteries.
- Enlarged right ventricle and right atrium.
- Increased pulmonary vasculature.
- 'Hilar dance' on fluoroscopy.

What are the ECG findings?

- Right bundle branch block pattern in ostium secundum type.
- Left axis deviation in ostium primum type.

What is the commonest arrhythmia seen in ASD?

Atrial fibrillation.

Victor Eisenmenger (1864–1932), German physician.
Rene Lutembacher, a French physician, described the Lutembacher syndrome in 1916.
Mary Holt, cardiologist, King's College Hospital, London.
Samuel Oram, cardiologist, King's College Hospital, London.

References

Borow, KM & Karp, R (1990) Atrial septal defect – lessons from the past, directions for the future. *N Engl J Med* **323:** 1698.
Campbell, M (1970) Natural history of atrial septal defect. *Br Heart J* **32:** 820–826.
Craig, JR & Selzer, A (1968) Natural history and prognosis of atrial septal defect. *Circulation* **37:** 805.
Holt, M & Oram, S (1960) Familial heart disease with skeletal malformation. *Br Heart J* **22:** 236.
Lutembacher, R (1916) De la stenose mitrale avec communication interauriculaire. *Arch Mal Coeur* **9:** 237.
Murphy, JG, Gersh, BJ, McGoon, MD et al (1990) Long term outcome after surgical repair of isolated atrial septal defect: follow up at 27 to 32 years. *N Engl J Med* **323:** 1645–1650.
Rocchini, AP (1990) Transcatheter closure of atrial septal defects: past, present and future. *Circulation* **82:** 1044–1045.

Case 21	Hypertrophic Obstructive Cardiomyopathy

Instruction

Examine this patient's cardiovascular system.

Salient features

- Carotid pulse is bifid.
- 'a' wave in the JVP.
- *Double apical impulse* (left ventricular heave with a prominent pre-systolic impulse).

- Pansystolic murmur at the apex and ejection systolic murmur along the left sternal border – accentuated by standing and Valsalva manoeuvre, fourth heart sound.

- Tell the examiner that you would like to take a family history of the following:
  Sudden death.
  Similar cardiomyopathy.

Questions

How may such a patient present?

- Dyspnoea.
- Syncope and sudden death.
- Angina pectoris.
- Palpitations.

What single investigation would you do to confirm your diagnosis?

Echocardiographic and the features are as follows:

- Asymmetrical septal hypertrophy (ASH).
- Systolic anterior motion of the mitral valve (SAM) and mitral regurgitation using Doppler ultrasound.

How would you manage such a patient?

Treatment is directed towards the following:

- Relief of symptoms.
- Prevention of arrhythmias and sudden death by administration of amiodarone.
- Improvement of ventricular function using beta blocker (propranolol up to 640 mg per day), verapamil, amiodarone, diuretics.
- Prevention of infective endocarditis.

- Surgery – such as myotomy or myectomy – relieves symptoms but does not alter the natural history of the disease.

What is the most characteristic pathophysiological abnormality in hypertrophic cardiomyopathy?

Diastolic dysfunction.

What ECG abnormalities may be seen?

- ST segment and T wave abnormalities.
- Tall R waves due to left ventricular hypertrophy.

- Prominent abnormal Q waves in the inferior and lateral leads (in 20% of cases).

Which condition has the most common association with hypertrophic obstructive cardiomyopathy?

Friedreich's ataxia.

John Goodwin, contemporary Emeritus Professor of Cardiology, Hammersmith Hospital, London.
Robert Roberts, Chief of Cardiology, Baylor School of Medicine, Houston, USA, whose chief interest is molecular biology.

References

Maron, BJ, Bonow, RO, Cannon III, RW et al (1987) Hypertrophic cardiomyopathy. Interrelations of clinical manifestations, pathophysiology and therapy. *N Engl J Med* **316**: 780, 844.
Morrow, AG & Braunwald, E (1959) Functional aortic stenosis. A malformation characterised by resistance to left ventricular outflow without anatomic obstruction. *Circulation* **20**: 181.
Teare, RD (1958) Asymmetrical hypertrophy of the heart in young adults. *Br Heart J* **20**: 1.

Case 22   Patent Ductus Arteriosus

Instruction

Examine this patient's heart.
Examine this patient's cardiovascular system.

Salient features

- Collapsing pulse.
- Heaving apex beat.

- Loud, continuous 'machinery' murmur, i.e. pansystolic and extending into early diastole – known as Gibson murmur, along the left upper sternal border, outer border of clavicle.

- Tell the examiner that you would like to take a maternal history of rubella.

Questions

Mention a few causes of a collapsing pulse.

Hyperdynamic circulation due to:

- Aortic regurgitation.
- Thyrotoxicosis.
- Severe anaemia.
- Paget's disease.
- Complete heart block.

■ Mention a few causes of continuous murmurs.

- Venous hum.
- Mitral regurgitant murmur with aortic regurgitant murmur.
- VSD with aortic regurgitation.
- Pulmonary arteriovenous fistula.
- Rupture of sinus of Valsalva.
- Coronary arteriovenous fistula.
- Bronchopulmonary artery anastomotic connection.
- Arteriovenous anastomoses of intercostal vessels following a fractured rib.

How would you investigate this patient?

- ECG may be normal or shows left ventricular hypertrophy.
- CXR may be normal, or there may be left ventricular and left atrial enlargement.
- Cardiac catheterisation establishes the presence and severity of the shunt.
- Angiography defines its anatomy.

What are the complications?

- Congestive cardiac failure is the commonest complication.
- Infective endocarditis or endarteritis.
- Pulmonary hypertension and reversal of shunt (causes differential cyanosis and clubbing, i.e. toes – *not* fingers – are clubbed and cyanosed).

How would you manage such patients?

- Within 1–3 weeks of birth: administer prostaglandin E synthesis inhibitor such as indomethacin.
- Children or adults with large shunts: perform surgery, i.e. ligation or division of the patent ductus arteriosus.

Note. Pulmonary hypertension is a contraindication for surgery.

Collapsing pulse is also called Corrigan's pulse after Sir Dominic J Corrigan (1802–1880), a Dublin born physician who graduated from Edinburgh.

References

Campbell, M (1968) Natural history of persistent ductus arteriosus. *Br Heart J* **30**: 4.
Gibson, GA (1990) Persistence of the arterial duct and its diagnosis. *Edin Med J* **8**: 1.
Heymann, MA, Rudolph, AM & Silverman, NH (1976) Closure of the ductus arteriosus by prostaglandin inhibition. *N Engl J Med* **295**: 530.
Krovetz, LJ & Rowe, RD (1972) Patent ductus, prematurity and pulmonary disease. *N Engl J Med* **287**: 513.

Case 23	Pulmonary Stenosis

Instruction

Examine this patient's heart

Salient features

- Normal pulse.
- Prominent 'a' wave in the JVP.

- Left parasternal heave.
- Ejection click (a valvular stenosis).
- Ejection systolic murmur in the upper left sternal border, best heard on inspiration, and a soft P_2.

- Tell the examiner that you would like to look for the following:
  Central cyanosis – indicating Fallot's tetralogy.
  VSD.
  ASD.
- Tell the examiner that you would like to ask for a history of maternal rubella.

Questions

What is the underlying cause of pulmonary stenosis?

- Congenital (commonest cause).
- Carcinoid tumour of small bowel.

What are the radiological findings?

- Normal aortic knuckle.
- Normal or enlarged pulmonary conus (due to poststenotic dilatation of a valvular stenosis).
- Large right atrium.

What are the complications of this condition?

- Cardiac failure.
- Infective endocarditis: blood cultures are rarely positive; the emboli are entirely in the pulmonary circulation and not systemic.

What are the types of pulmonary stenosis?

- Valvular.
- Subvalvular – infundibular and subinfundibular.
- Supravalvular.

Do you know of any eponymous syndromes linked to pulmonary stenosis?

- Noonan's syndrome: short stature, ptosis, downward slanting eyes, wide-spaced eyes (hypertelorism), low-set ears, webbed neck, mental retardation, low posterior hairline and pulmonary stenosis.
- Watson's syndrome: café-au-lait spots, mental retardation and pulmonary stenosis.

References

Abrahams DG & Wood, P (1951) Pulmonary stenosis with normal aortic root. *Br Heart J* **13**: 519.
Mody, MR (1975) The natural history of uncomplicated valvular pulmonic stenosis. *Am Heart J* **90**: 317.

Case 24	Dextrocardia

Instruction

Examine this patient's precordium.
Listen to this patient's heart.

Salient features

- Apex beat is absent on the left side and present on the right.
- Heart sounds are better heard on the right side of the chest.

- Tell the examiner that you would like to perform the following checks:
  Ascertain whether the liver dullness is present on the right or left side.
  Examine the chest for bronchiectasis.
  Obtain a CXR (look for right-sided gastric bubble).
  Obtain an ECG (inversion of all complexes in lead I).

Questions

What is Kartagener's syndrome?

A type of immotile cilia syndrome in which there is dextrocardia or situs inversus, bronchiectasis and dysplasia of the frontal sinuses.

Which other abnormality has been associated with dextrocardia?

Asplenia (blood smear may show Heinz bodies, Howell–Jolly bodies).

What do you understand by the term 'situs inversus'?

Right cardiac apex, right stomach, right-sided descending aorta.

What do you understand by the term 'dextroversion'?

Right-sided cardiac apex, left-sided stomach, left-sided descending aorta.

What do you understand by the term 'levoversion'?

Left-sided apex, right-sided stomach and right descending aorta.

M Kartagener (b, 1897), a Swiss physician, described this condition in 1933.

References

Kartagener M (1933) Zür pathogenese der Bronchiektasien; Bronchiektasien bei Situs Viscerum Inversus. *Beitr Klin Tuberk* **83**: 489.

Katz, M, Denzier, EE, Nangeroni, L & Sussman, D (1950) Kartagener's syndrome (situs inversus, bronchiectasis and chronic sinusitis). *N Engl J Med* **240**. 730.

Rose, V, Izukawa, I & Moes CAF (1975) Syndromes of asplenia and polysplenia. A review of cardiac and non-cardiac malformations in 60 cases with special reference to diagnosis and prognosis. *Br Heart J* **37**: 840.

Case 25	Coarctation of Aorta

Instruction

Examine this patient's cardiovascular system.

Salient features

- The upper torso is better developed than the lower part.

- Scapular collaterals are visible (listen over these collaterals).
- Radial pulse on left side may be less prominent.
- Heaving apex due to left ventricular hypertrophy.
- Short systolic murmur is present in the chest and back (there may also be an ejection systolic murmur of bicuspid aortic stenotic valve or continuous murmur of a patent ductus arteriosus).
- Radiofemoral delay (simultaneous palpation of the brachial and femoral arteries using the thumbs is the most convenient method of comparing pulsations in the upper and lower limbs).

- Tell the examiner that you would like to look for the following:
  Marfan's syndrome (arm span greater than height);
  Turner's syndrome (webbing of neck, increasing carrying angle);
  Berry aneurysms (extraocular movements impaired due to third cranial nerve involvement).

Questions

What radiological findings may be seen in such a patient?

- Poststenotic dilatation of the aorta.
- Dilated left subclavian artery high on the left mediastinal border.
- Rib notching.

What causes rib notching?

Collateral flow through dilated, tortuous and pulsatile posterior intercostal arteries typically causes notching on the undersurfaces of the posterior portions of the ribs. The anterior parts of the ribs are spared because the anterior intercostal arteries do not run in costal grooves. Notching is seldom found above the third or below the ninth rib and rarely appears before the age of 6 years.

Mention a few conditions where rib notching is seen.

- Coarctation of aorta
- Pulmonary oligaemia.
- Blalock–Taussig shunt.
- Subclavian artery obstruction.

- Superior vena caval obstruction.
- Neurofibromatosis.
- Arteriovenous malformations of the lung or chest wall.

At what age does this condition manifest?

It is particularly likely to produce significant symptoms in early infancy (presents as cardiac failure) or between the ages of 20 and 30 years.

How would you manage this patient?

- FBC, urea and electrolytes.
- CXR, ECG.
- Echocardiogram.
- Cardiac catheterisation and aortic and coronary angiogram.

What are the complications of aortic coarctation?

- Severe hypertension and resulting complications:
    Stroke.
    Left ventricular failure.
    Rupture of aorta.
- Infective endocarditis.

What are the fundal findings in coarctation of the aorta?

Hypertension due to coarctation of aorta causes retinal arteries to be tortuous with frequent 'U' turns and, curiously, the classical signs of hypertensive retinopathy are rarely seen.

What is the treatment of such patients?

Surgical resection and end to end anastomosis, although a tubular graft may be required if the narrowed segment is too long.

| Case 26 | Eisenmenger Syndrome |

Instruction

Examine this patient's heart.
Examine this patient's cardiovascular system.

Salient features

- Clubbing of fingers and central cyanosis.

- 'a' waves in the JVP, 'v' wave if tricuspid regurgitation is also present.
- Left parasternal heave, palpable P_2.
- Loud P_2, pulmonary ejection click, early diastolic murmur of pulmonary regurgitation (Graham Steell murmur).
- Loud pansystolic murmur of tricuspid regurgitation.

- The clinical findings with an associated defect are as follows:
    VSD – single second sound.
    ASD – fixed, wide split second sound.
    Patent ductus arteriosus – reverse split of second sound and differential cyanosis where lower-limb cyanosis is marked.

Questions

What do you understand by Eisenmenger syndrome?

Pulmonary hypertension with a reversed or bidirectional shunt and it matters very little where the shunt happens to be (e.g. VSD, ASD, patent ductus arteriosus, persistent truncus arteriosus, single ventricle or common atrioventricular canal).

What do you understand by Eisenmenger complex?

Eisenmenger complex is a VSD with a right-to-left shunt in the absence of pulmonary stenosis.

Mention some cyanotic heart diseases seen in infancy.

Tetralogy of Fallot, Transposition of the great vessels, Tricuspid atresia, Total anomalous pulmonary venous connection.

What is the age of onset of Eisenmenger syndrome?

In the case of patent ductus arteriosus and VSD about 80% occur in infancy, whereas in the case of ASD over 90% occur in adult life.

What are the symptoms of Eisenmenger syndrome?

Angina, syncope, haemoptysis and congestive cardiac failure.

What are the radiological features of Eisenmenger syndrome?

- Conspicuous dilatation of the pulmonary artery with slight to moderate enlargement of the heart (predominantly right ventricle).
- Peripheral markings are oligaemic.

How do these patients succumb?

- Haemoptysis.
- Cerebral abscess.
- Bacterial endocarditis.
- Heart failure.
- Cerebral thrombosis.

Victor Eisenmenger was a German physician who described this condition in an infant in 1897. His patient had cyanosis since infancy and had a fairly good quality of life until he succumbed at the age of 32.

References

Steell, G (1888) The murmur of high pressure in the pulmonary artery. *Med Chron* (Manchester) **9**: 182–188.
Wood, P (1958) The Eisenmenger syndrome. *Br Med J* **2**: 701, 709.

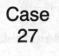

Case 27   Fallot's Tetralogy

Instruction

Examine this patient's heart.

Salient features

- Clubbing.
- Left radial pulse is not as prominent as the right.
- Central cyanosis.
- Thoracotomy scar may be seen (indicating Blalock–Taussig shunt).
- Left parasternal heave.
- Ejection systolic murmur is heard in the pulmonary area.

Questions

What are the constituents of Fallot's tetralogy?

- VSD with a right-to-left shunt.
- Pulmonary stenosis (infundibular or valvular).
- Right ventricular hypertrophy.
- Dextroposition of the aorta with it overriding the septal defect.

How may a patient with Fallot's tetralogy present?

- Syncope (in 20% of cases).
- Squatting.
- Shortness of breath.
- Growth retardation.

What are complications of Fallot's tetralogy?

- Cyanotic and syncopal spells.
- Cerebral abscess (in 10% of cases).
- Endocarditis (in 10% of cases).
- Strokes – thrombotic secondary to polycythaemia.
- Paradoxical emboli.

What do you understand by a Blalock–Taussig shunt?

It is the anastomosis of the left subclavian artery to the left pulmonary artery with the intention to increase pulmonary blood flow.

Why is it less frequently seen in adults in the recent past?

With ready availability of cardiopulmonary bypass, such patients have total correction of their anomalies at an early age.

What is Fallot's trilogy?

ASD, pulmonary stenosis and right ventricular hypertrophy.

What is Fallot's pentalogy?

Fallot's tetralogy with associated ASD is known as Fallot's pentalogy.

What conditions are associated with Fallot's tetralogy?

- Right-sided aortic arch (in 30% of cases).
- Double aortic arch.
- Left-sided superior vena cava (in 10% of cases).
- ASD.

Mention the common congenital heart diseases.

VSD, ASD of the secundum type, patent ductus arteriosus and Fallot's tetralogy are the common congenital heart diseases in order of frequency.

What are the CXR findings?

- Boot-shaped heart.
- Enlarged right ventricle.
- Decreased pulmonary vasculature.
- Right-sided aortic arch (in 30% of cases).

Etienne-Louis Arthur Fallot (1850–1911), Professor of Hygiene and Legal Medicine in Marseilles, published his *Contribution to the pathologic anatomy of morbus coeruleus cardiac cyanosis* in 1888. The tetralogy was first described by N Stensen, Professor of Anatomy in Copenhagen, in 1672.
Helen Brook Taussing (1898–1986) is the founder of American paediatric cardiology and she collaborated with Alfred Blalock (1899–1964) in the development of palliative surgery for Fallot's tetralogy.

References

Higgins, CB & Mulder, DG (1972) Tetralogy of Fallot in the adult. *Am J Cardiol* **28:** 837.

NEUROLOGY

Examination of the Cranial Nerves

First cranial nerve

- Ask the patient, 'Have you noticed any change in your sense of smell recently?'
- If the examiner requires you to test the sense of smell use an odour which can be readily identified, such as soap or clove oil.

Second cranial nerve

- First check visual acuity using a pocket Snellen's chart and finger counting.
- Make sure that the patient wears his or her spectacles should he or she use them.
- Check visual fields using a hat pin; your instructions to the patient should be clear and precise.
- Comment on the pupils (size, shape, inequality) and test their reaction to light (direct and indirect reaction) and to accommodation.
- Examine the fundus.

Third, fourth and sixth cranial nerves

- Test eye movements (remember to ask the patient whether he or she sees a double image).
- Remember to comment on nystagmus.
- Comment on ptosis if present (seen in third nerve palsy).

Fifth cranial nerve

- Test the masseters – 'Clench your teeth' – taking care to palpate the muscles.

- Test the pterygoids – 'Open your mouth' – and note that the jaw deviates to the side of lesion.
- Test corneal sensation and facial sensation using cotton wool.
- Test the jaw jerk.

Seventh cranial nerve

Remember that the facial nerve is a motor nerve.
- Ask the patient, 'Show me your teeth'.
- Ask the patient, 'Screw your eyes tightly shut and don't let me open them'.

Eighth cranial nerve

- Occlude each external auditory meatus with your finger and whisper short phrases, asking the patient to repeat them.
- Perform Rinne's and Weber's tests (use a tuning fork with a frequency of 256 cycles per second (c.p.s.).

Ninth and tenth cranial nerves

- Ask the patient, 'Open your mouth and say "aah" '; observe the soft palate using a torch (the soft palate is pulled to the normal side on saying 'aah').
- Tell the examiner that you would like to check for gag reflex.

Eleventh cranial nerve

- Ask the patient, 'Shrug your shoulders', and try to push them down simultaneously (this tests the trapezii muscles).
- Test the sternomastoids.

Twelfth cranial nerve

- Ask the patient, 'Open your mouth'; comment on fasciculations of the tongue while in the mouth. Comment on wasting.
- Ask the patient, 'Stick your tongue out' (it deviates to the side of the lesion).

HA Rinnie (1819–1868), German ear, nose and throat physician.
FE Weber-Liel (1832–1891), German otologist.

Neurological Examination of the Patient's Upper Limbs

1. *Introduce* yourself to the patient and ask him to take his top things off so that both his arms are well exposed. If the patient is female cover her breasts with suitable clothing so that she is decent.

2. *Comment on wasting, tremor, fasciculations.*

3. *Assess tone*: 'Let your arms go loose and let me move them for you'.
   - Flex and extend the wrists passively – cogwheel rigidity may be elicited by this method.
   - Flex and extend at the elbows, pronate and supinate at the forearm – lead pipe rigidity and clasp knife spasticity may be elicited by these methods.

4. *Test power*: 'I am going to test the strength of the muscles of your arms'.
   - Tell the patient, 'Hold your arms stretched out in front of you and then close your eyes'. Observe for drift, action tremor.
   - Shoulder abduction: 'Hold your arms outwards at your sides (like this) and keep them up; don't let me stop you'. Chief movers are the deltoids, C5. (**Note.** Supraspinatus is responsible for the initiation of abduction and is responsible for the first 60 degrees of this movement. However, this method of testing only assesses the power of the deltoids.)
   - Shoulder adduction: 'Push your arms in towards you and don't let me stop you'. Chief movers are the pectoral muscles, C6–8.
   - Elbow flexion: 'Bend your elbows and pull me towards you; don't let me stop you'. Chief mover is the biceps, C5.
   - Elbow extension: 'Straighten your elbow and push me away; don't let me stop you'. Chief mover is the triceps, C7.
   - Wrist extension: 'Clench your fist and cock your wrists up; don't let me stop you'. Chief mover is C7.
   - Wrist flexion: 'Now push the other way'. Chief mover is C7.
   - Finger abduction: 'Spread your fingers wide apart and don't let me push them together'. Chief movers are the dorsal interossei, T1 (ulnar nerve). **Note. D**orsal interossei **ab**duct: mnemonic, DAB.
   - Finger adduction: 'Hold this piece of paper between your fingers and don't let me snatch it away'. Chief movers are the palmar interossei, T1 (ulnar nerve). **Note. P**almar interossei **ad**duct: mnemonic, PAD.
   - Thumb adduction: 'Hold your palms facing the ceiling and now point your thumb towards the ceiling; don't let me stop you'.

Chief mover is the abductor pollicis brevis, C8, T1 (median nerve).
- Flexion of the fingers: 'Grip these two fingers of mine tightly and don't let them go.' Chief movers are the long and short flexors of the fingers, C8.

Note

- The median nerve supplies the lateral two lumbricals, opponens pollicis, abductor pollicis brevis, flexor pollicis brevis: mnemonic, LOAF.
- The ulnar nerve supplies all other small muscles of the hand.
- The lumbricals are responsible for flexion at the metacarpophalangeal joint when the interphalangeal joints are in extension.
- Power is graded from 0 to 5:
    0, Absence of movement.
    1, Flicker of movement on voluntary contraction.
    2, Movement present when gravity is eliminated.
    3, Movement against gravity but not against resistance.
    4, Movement against resistance but not full strength.
    5, Normal power.
5. *Test deep tendon reflexes*: biceps, C5, C6; triceps, C7; supinator, C5, C6.
- Biceps, C5, C6.
- Triceps, C7.
- Supinator, C5, C6.
- If the reflexes are absent, test after reinforcement – ask the patient to clench his or her teeth.
- *Inversion of the supinator reflex*. When the supinator jerk is elicited the normal response is a slight flexion of the fingers, contraction of the brachioradialis and flexion at the elbow joint. The jerk is said to be 'inverted' when finger flexion is the sole response, with contraction of the brachioradialis and elbow flexion being absent. There is associated absence of the biceps jerk and exaggeration of the triceps jerk.
    The inverted jerk indicates a lower motor neuron lesion at the fifth cervical level and an upper motor neuron lesion below this level. It could be due to cervical spondylosis, trauma to cervical cord, spinal cord tumours at this level and syringomyelia.
6. *Test co-ordination*
- Finger–note–finger test: 'Touch your nose with your index finger and now touch my finger'.
- Rapid alternating movement of one hand over the other.
7. *Test sensation*
- Light touch: use cotton wool and check each dermatome.
- Pinprick: demonstrate first the sharp end and then the blunt end

on the sternum; then check each dermatome for sharp or blunt sensation with the eyes closed.
- Joint position sense: check in the distal interphalangeal joint of the thumb.
- Vibration sense: use a tuning fork of 128 c.p.s. First test on the sternum so that the patient can recognise the vibration and then check over the fingers and moving proximally if vibration sense is absent distally.

Remember:
- Joint sense and vibration sense are carried in the dorsal columns.
- Pain and temperature are carried in the lateral spinothalamic tracts.
- Light touch is carried in both the above tracts.

Neurological Examination of the Patient's Lower Limbs

1. *Introduce* yourself and then ensure that the lower limbs are well exposed. At the same time it is important to ensure that the patient is decent – cover the genital area with a towel or any suitable clothing.
2. *Inspect for wasting, fasciculations* (tap the muscles of the leg and thigh to elicit fasciculations if not seen).
3. *Assess tone*
   - Ask the patient, 'Let your leg go loose and lax and let me move it for you'; then passively flex and extend the leg at the knee and hip.
   - Roll the extended leg, feeling for resistance.
   - Put your hand behind the knee and pull it upwards, observing the foot to check whether or not it flops.
   - If there is spasticity or increased tone then test for ankle clonus and patellar clonus.
4. *Test power* (begin at the hips): 'I am going to test the strength of the muscles of your legs'.
   - Hip flexion: 'Lift your leg straight up and keep it there; don't let me stop you'. Chief mover is the iliopsoas L1, L2.
   - Hip extension: 'Push your leg downwards into your bed and don't let me stop you'. Chief movers are the glutei, L4, L5.
   - Hip abduction: 'Push your thigh out against my hand'. Chief movers are the glutei, L4, L5.
   - Hip adduction: 'Push your thigh inwards against my hand'. Chief movers are the adductors of the thigh, L2–4.

- Knee flexion: 'Bend your knee and pull your heel towards you; don't let me stop you'. Chief movers are the hamstrings, L5, S1.
- Knee extension: 'Straighten your knee and don't let me stop you'. Chief movers are the quadriceps, L3, L4.
- Plantar flexion of the ankle: 'Push your foot downwards against my hand'. Chief mover is the gastrocnemius, S1.
- Dorsiflexion of the ankle: 'Move your foot up and don't let me stop you'. Chief movers are the tibialis anterior and long extensors, L4, L5.
- Inversion of the foot: 'Push your foot inwards against my hand'. Chief movers are the tibialis anterior and posterior, L4.
- Eversion of the foot: 'Push your foot outwards against my hand'. Chief movers are the peronei, S1.
- Extension of the great toe: 'Pull your toe upwards and don't let me stop you'. Chief mover is the extensor hallucis longus, L5.

5. *Test the plantar response*: 'I am going to tickle the bottom of your foot and use an orange stick to stimulate the outer portion of the sole'. Always describe the response as either downgoing or upgoing.

    Remember that if the feet are cold (when outside the bed-clothes for long) the response may be equivocal.

6. *Test deep tendon reflexes*
   - Knee jerk, L4.
   - Ankle jerk, S1.
   - If absent, reinforce by asking the patient to pull outwards his clasped hands. Do not tie your arms into a knot while testing the left ankle jerk from the patient's right hand side. Avoid jabbing the patient while eliciting reflexes.

7. *Test co-ordination*
   - Heel–shin test.

8. *Test sensation*
   - Light touch.
   - Pinprick.
   - Joint position sense – hold the lateral aspect of the big toe while eliciting this.
   - Vibration sense.

   Note. When there is weakness of the limbs tell the examiner that you would like to check sensation in the sacral area.

9. *Romberg's test*: 'Please stand up with your legs together and now close your eyes'. Take care to protect the patient if he or she sways and tends to fall.

10. *Check gait* and if heel–shin test is affected then test tandem walking (ask the patient to walk along a straight line with one heel in front of the other foot).

JJ Babinski (1857–1932), of Polish origin, graduated from University of Paris with a thesis on multiple sclerosis. Babinski response refers to upgoing plantars in upper motor neuron lesions. He described adiposogenitalis a year before Frolich.

| Case 28 | Bilateral Spastic Paralysis (Spastic Paraplegia) |

Instruction

Carry out a neurological examination of this patient's lower limbs.

Salient features

- Increased tone in both lower limbs.
- Hyperreflexia.
- Ankle clonus.
- Weakness in both lower limbs.

- Remember to check the sensory level and examine the spine.
- If permitted to examine the upper arms it may be possible to localise the lesion using the deep tendon reflexes – an absent biceps and a brisk supinator jerk (inversion of the supinator jerk) or an absent biceps and supinator with a brisk triceps jerk localises the lesion to C5/C6.
- Tell the examiner that you would like to do the following:
   Ask about bladder symptoms and check sacral sensation.
   Ask whether the weakness was sudden or gradual.
   Check for wasted hands (cervical spondylosis, motor neuron disease, syringomyelia).
   Check for cerebellar signs (multiple sclerosis, Friedreich's ataxia).
   Take a history of birth anoxia (cerebral palsy).

Questions

What is your differential diagnosis?

- Cord compression.
- Multiple sclerosis.

- Traumatic (especially motor vehicle accidents).
- Motor neuron disease.
- Transverse myelitis.
- Syringomyelia.
- Subacute combined degeneration of the cord (peripheral neuropathy).
- Anterior spinal artery thrombosis.

- Tabes dorsalis.
- Friedreich's ataxia.
- Familial spastic paraplegia.

What intracranial cause for spastic paraparesis do you know?

Parasagittal falx meningioma.

What investigations would you do?

- Myelogram.
- Check cerebrospinal fluid (CSF) for oligoclonal bands.
- Serum vitamin B_{12} levels.

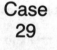

Case 29   Hemiplegia

Instruction

Carry out a neurological examination of this patient.

Salient features

- Unilateral upper motor neuron seventh nerve palsy.

- Weakness of the upper and lower limbs on the same side with upper motor neuron signs – increased tone, hyperreflexia and upgoing plantar response.
- Do not forget sensory signs, in particular joint sensation which is important in rehabilitation.

- Examine:
   For homonymous hemianopia and sensory inattention.
   For carotid bruits.
   For speech defects.
   The pulse for atrial fibrillation.
   The heart for murmurs.
- Tell the examiner that you would like to check the blood pressure and check the urine for sugar.

Questions

What is your diagnosis?

- This patient has had a stroke causing a right or left hemiplegia and the underlying cause is a vascular event such as thrombosis, embolism or haemorrhage.
- Neoplasm in the brain.

How would you manage such a patient?

- FBC, ESR.
- Urine sugar.
- ECG.
- CXR.
- Computerised tomography (CT) scan, echocardiography, carotid digital subtraction angiography (DSA) in selected patients.
- Physiotherapy and speech therapy assessment.
- Control of risk factors – diabetes, hypertension, hyperlipidaemia, stop smoking, stop oral contraceptives.

How would you manage a patient with TIA?

- Stop smoking.
- Aspirin.
- Duplex ultrasound of the carotid vessels.
- Carotid artery DSA.

What do you understand by the term 'TIA'?

An acute loss of focal cerebral or ocular function with symptoms lasting less than 24 h.

Why is it important to differentiate a carotid TIA from a vertebrobasilar TIA?

Carotid TIAs may be amenable to surgery. Furthermore, a TIA in the anterior circulation is generally of more serious prognostic significance than a TIA in the posterior circulation.

What are the features of a carotid TIA?

Hemiparesis, aphasia or transient loss of vision in one eye only (amaurosis fugax).

What are the features of a vertebrobasilar TIA?

- Vertigo, dysphagia, ataxia and drop attacks (at least two of these should occur together).
- Bilateral or alternating weakness or sensory symptoms.
- Sudden bilateral blindness in patients aged over 40.

What are the clinical features that would interest you for the rehabilitation of a stroke?

- Independence in the activities of daily living – bathing, dressing, toileting, transferring, continence and feeding.
- Independence in more complex activities such as meal preparation, shopping, financial management, housekeeping, transportation, medication-taking and laundering.

What are the causes of stroke in the young?

- Embolism (look for underlying valvular heart disease, atrial fibrillation).
- Connective tissue disorder.
- Luetic disease (neurosyphilis).
- Intracranial infection: look for underlying acquired immune deficiency syndrome (AIDS), otitis media, cyanotic heart disease.

What are the risk factors for stroke?

Hypertension, ischaemic heart disease, atrial fibrillation, peripheral vascular disease, diabetes, smoking, previous TIA, cervical bruit, hyperlipidaemia, raised haematocrit, oral contraceptive pill, cardiomyopathy.

Why is it important to treat TIA?

Prospective studies have shown that within 5 years following a TIA:
    One out of six patients will have suffered a stroke.
    One out of four patients will have died (either of a stroke or heart disease).

■ What is the role of carotid endarterectomy in patients with a carotid TIA?

- For patients with severe stenosis (70–99%) the risks of surgery were significantly outweighed by the later benefits.
- For patients with mild stenosis (0–29% of cases) there was little 3-year risk of ipsilateral ischaemic stroke, even in the absence of surgery, so that any 3-year benefits of surgery were small and were outweighed by its early risks.
- For patients with moderate stenosis (30–69% of cases) the balance of surgical risk and eventual benefit is still being evaluated.

What do you understand by the term 'RIND'?

Reversible ischaemic neurological disease, in which the symptoms and signs reverse within a week but not within 24 hours.

What are lacunar infarcts?

Lacunar infarcts are seen in hypertensives and consist of small infarcts in the region of internal capsule (causing partial hemiparesis or hemisensory impairment), pons (ataxia of cerebellar type, partial hemiparesis), basal ganglia or thalamus. They are often multiple. Lacunae are thought to be caused by occlusion of small branch arteries or by rupture of Charcot–Bouchard microaneurysms producing a small haematoma which resolves, leaving an area of infarction.

What are the criteria for brain death?

- Absent brain stem function – fixed dilated pupils, absent corneal and gag reflexes, absent caloric responses, lack of spontaneous respiration.
- Absent cortical function – deep coma.
- A known untreatable cause such as cardiac arrest, intracerebral haemorrhage, trauma.

Charles Warlow, Professor of Neurosciences, Edinburgh.

References

Barnett, HJM (1991) Beneficial effect of carotid endarterectomy in symptomatic patients with high-grade carotid stenosis – North American Symptomatic Carotid Endarterectomy Trial Collaborators. *N Engl J Med* **325**: 445–453.
Kistler, JP, Buonanno, FS & Gress, DR (1991) Carotid endarterectomy – specific therapy based on pathophysiology. *N Engl J Med* **325**: 505.
Sandercock, PAG (1991) Recent developments in the diagnosis and management of

patients with transient ischaemic attacks and minor ischaemic strokes. *Q J Med* **286:** 101–112.

Warlow, C (1991) European Carotid Surgery Trial: interim results for symptomatic patients with severe (70–99%) or patients with mild (0–29%) carotid stenosis. *Lancet* **337:** 1235.

Case 30	Ptosis and Horner's Syndrome

Salient features

In the examination if you notice ptosis then you must answer the following questions:

- Is ptosis complete or incomplete?
- Is ptosis unilateral or bilateral?
- Is the pupil constricted (Horner's syndrome) or dilated (third nerve palsy)?
- Are extraocular movements involved (third nerve palsy or myasthenia gravis)?
- Is the eyeball sunken or not (enophthalmos)?
- Is the light reflex intact (intact light reflex in Horner's syndrome)?

If the patient has Horner's syndrome then quickly proceed as follows:

- Examine the supraclavicular area:
  Percuss supraclavicular area, looking for dullness of Pancoast's tumour.
  Look for scar of cervical sympathectomy (be prepared with indications for cervical sympathectomy).
  Look for enlarged lymph nodes.
- Examine the neck:
  For carotid and aortic aneurysms.
  For tracheal deviation (Pancoast's tumour).
- Examine the hands:
  For small muscle wasting.
  For pain sensation with a pin.
  For clubbing.

These should help in making a diagnosis of syringomyelia or Pancoast's tumour.

- Tell the examiner that you would like to ask the patient whether or not there is an absence of sweating on one side of the face.
- If there is no clue so far about the cause then tell the examiner you would like to examine for nystagmus, cerebellar signs, cranial nerves, pale discs and pyramidal signs to ascertain brain stem vascular disease or demyelination.

Questions

What causes Horner's syndrome?

The syndrome is due to the involvement of the sympathetic pathway. It starts in the sympathetic nucleus and travels through the brain stem and spinal cord to the level of C8/T1/T2 to the sympathetic chain, stellate ganglion and carotid sympathetic plexus.

What additional feature would you see in congenital Horner's syndrome?

There would be heterochromia of the iris, i.e. the iris remains grey-blue.

How would you determine the level of lesion using only the history?

The level of lesion is determined by the distribution of the loss of sweating:

- Central lesion – sweating over the entire half of the head, arm and upper trunk is lost.
- Lesions of the neck:
  Proximal to the superior cervical ganglion – diminished sweating on the face.
  Distal to the superior cervical ganglion – sweating is not affected.

How would you differentiate whether the lesion is above the superior ganglion (peripheral) or below the superior cervical ganglion (central)?

Test	Above	Below
Sweating	Such lesions may not affect sweating at all as the main outflow to the facial blood vessels is below the superior cervical ganglion	Such lesions usually affect sweating over the entire head, neck, arm and upper trunk. Lesions in the lower neck affect sweating over the entire face

Test	Above	Below
Cocaine 4% in both eyes	Dilates the normal pupil No effect on affected side	Dilates both pupils
Adrenaline 1:1000 in both eyes	Dilates affected eye No effect on normal side	No effect on both sides

Note. In peripheral lesions there is depletion of amine oxidase due to postganglionic denervation. As a result this sensitises the pupil to 1:10 000 adrenaline whereas it has no effect on the normal pupil or in central lesions (where the presence of the enzyme rapidly destroys the adrenaline).

Mention one cause of intermittent Horner's syndrome.

Migraine.

What are the causes of ptosis?

- Unilateral:
    Third nerve palsy.
    Horner's syndrome.
    Myasthenia gravis.
    Congenital or idiopathic.
- Bilateral:
    Myasthenia gravis.
    Dystrophia myotonica.
    Ocular myopathy or oculopharyngeal muscular dystrophy.
  Congenital:
    Tabes dorsalis.
    Bilateral Horner's syndrome (as in syringomyelia).

If this patient has a Pancoast's tumour what is the most likely underlying pathology?

Squamous cell carcinoma.

JF Horner (1831–1886), Professor of Ophthalmology in Zurich. Horner himself conceded that Claude Bernard had recognised the syndrome before him.
Henry K Pancoast (1875–1939), the first Professor of Radiology in the US at the University of Pennsylvania.

Case 31	Argyll Robertson Pupil

Instruction

Examine this patient's eyes.

Salient features

- The pupils are small and irregular.
- Light reflex is absent.
- Accommodation reflex is intact.
- There may be depigmentation of the iris.

- Tell the examiner that you would like to do the following:
    Examine for vibration and position sense.
    Test Romberg's sign and deep tendon reflexes (decreased).
    Ask the patient about lancinating pains.
    Check syphilitic serology.
    Check urine for sugar.
- Remember that these pupils show little response to atropine, physostigmine or methacholine.

Questions

What are the causes of Argyll Robertson pupil?

- Neurosyphilis – tabes dorsalis.
- Diabetes mellitus.
- Pinealoma.
- Brain stem encephalitis.

Mention a few causes of a small pupil.

- Senile miosis.
- Pilocarpine drops in the treatment of glaucoma.

■ What is 'reversed' Argyll Robertson pupil?

The pupils react to light but not to accommodation – seen in Parkinsonism caused by encephalitis lethargica.

Douglas MCL Argyll Robertson (1837–1909) of Edinburgh described these pupils in 1869 in patients with neurosyphilis. His studies on the effects of the extracts of the Calabar bean (*Physostigma venomas*) on the pupil were widely acclaimed. He was the President of the Royal College of Surgeons of Edinburgh.

Case 32 | Holmes–Adie Syndrome

Instruction

Examine this patient's eyes.

Salient features

- The patient is usually a young woman.
- The pupil is large, regular and circular.
- The pupil will react sluggishly or fail to react to light.

  However, if a strong and persistent stimulus is used it can be shown that the pupil contracts excessively to a very small size and when the stimulus is removed it returns to its former size gradually – this is known as 'myotonic' pupil.

- Tell the examiner that you would like to check the ankle jerks and you expect them to be absent.

Questions

What is the significance of this condition?

It is benign and must not be mistaken for Argyll Robertson pupil.

What are the causes of a dilated pupil?

- Mydriatic eye drops.
- Third nerve lesion.

- Holmes–Adie syndrome.
- Lens implant, iridectomy.
- Deep coma, death.

What are the causes of a small pupil?

- Old age.
- Pilocarpine eye drops.
- Horner's syndrome.
- Argyll Robertson pupil.
- Pontine lesion.
- Narcotics.

How does the Holmes–Adie pupil react to 2.5% methacholine?

It usually constricts, indicating a supersensitivity to acetylcholine secondary to parasympathetic denervation resulting from degeneration of postganglionic neurons and neurons in the ciliary ganglion.

Which conditions may accompany this syndrome?

Dysautonomias such as:

- Ross's syndrome (segmental loss of sweating).
- Cardiac arrhythmias.

Sir Gordon M Holmes (1876–1965) and WJ Adie (1886–1935) were London neurologists who described the condition independently in 1931.

| Case 33 | Homonymous Hemianopia |

Instruction

Examine this patient's eyes.
Examine this patient's visual fields.

Salient features

- Homonymous hemianopia.

- Check visual acuity; examine the fundus.
- Tell the examiner that you would like to do a full neurological examination to look for an underlying cause:
    Stroke.
    Intracranial tumour.

Questions

Where is the lesion?

The lesion is in the optic tract and beyond (visual acuity is intact when the macula is spared).

What further investigations would you do?

- Formal field testing: perimetry is particularly important if the patient holds a driver's licence.
- CT head scan.

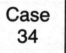

Case 34   Bitemporal Hemianopia

Instruction

Examine this patient's eyes.
Examine this patient's visual fields.

Salient features

- Bitemporal hemianopia which is due to a lesion of the optic chiasma.

- Examine the hands and face for acromegaly.
- Tell the examiner that you would like to look for signs of hypopituitarism (see page 255). The probable causes are as follows:
  Pituitary tumour.
  Craniopharyngioma.
  Suprasellar meningioma.
  Aneurysms.
  Metastases.
  Glioma.

Questions

How would you investigate this patient?

- Formal field testing – perimetry.
- Skull X-ray (calcification of craniopharyngioma and size of pituitary fossa which is best seen in lateral skull X-ray).
- CT head scan.

Case 35	Central Scotoma

Instruction

Examine this patient's visual fields.

Salient features

- Central scotoma.
- Tell the examiner that you would like to examine the fundus.
- Remember that the optic discs may be:
  Pale (optic atrophy).
  Normal (retrobulbar neuritis).
  Swollen and pink (papillitis).

Questions

Mention a few underlying causes for central scotoma.

The differential diagnosis is as follows:
- Demyelinating disorders (multiple sclerosis).
- Optic nerve compression by tumour, aneurysm.
- Glaucoma.
- Toxins – methanol, tobacco, lead, arsenical poisoning.
- Ischaemic – including central retinal artery occlusion due to thromboembolism, temporal arteritis, idiopathic acute ischaemic optic neuropathy, syphilis.
- Hereditary disorders – Friedreich's ataxia, Leber's optic atrophy.
- Paget's disease.
- Vitamin B_{12} deficiency.
- Secondary to retinitis pigmentosa.

Case 36	Tunnel Vision

Instruction

Examine this patient's eyes.
Examine this patient's visual fields.

Salient features

- Intact central vision with constriction of the peripheral fields.
- Examine for the following:
  Retinitis pigmentosa (see page 372).
  Choroidoretinitis (see page 376).
  Glaucoma.

Case 37 | Parkinson's Syndrome

Instruction

Examine this patient.

Salient features

- Usually, florid cases are kept and the striking abnormalities are an expressionless face (mask-like), resting or pill-rolling movement and drooling of saliva.

  Proceed in a systematic manner:

- Comment on the expressionless face, pill rolling movement and drooling of saliva so that the examiner knows that you have observed these abnormalities. Elicit bradykinesia by asking the patient to touch his or her thumb with each finger in turn.
- Examine the tone, in particular at the wrist for cogwheel rigidity.
- Proceed to do the glabellar tap (tap the forehead just above the bridge of the nose repeatedly: in normal people the blinking will stop after a while whereas in Parkinson's the patient continues to blink. (It must be remembered that this is an unreliable sign.)
- Ask the patient to walk and comment on the paucity of movement including absence of arm swing and festinating gait (the patient walks with a stooped posture as if trying to catch up with his or her centre of gravity).

- Tell the examiner you would like to ask the patient a few questions with a view to assessing his or her speech and to elicit a drug history, particularly regarding neuroleptics.
- Tell the examiner that you would like to check the following:
  Blood pressure, both lying and standing (Shy–Drager syndrome – postural hypotension). Remember that L-dopa can cause postural hypotension.
  Extraocular movements (Steel–Richardson–Olzewski where vertical eye movements are impaired).
- Comment on seborrhoea if any.

Questions

What comprises Parkinson's syndrome?

The components of Parkinson's syndrome are as follows:
   Tremor
   Bradykinesia
   Rigidity.
   Loss of postural reflexes.

What are the causes of Parkinson's syndrome?

- Idiopathic degeneration of the substantia nigra (also known as Parkinson's disease).
- Drugs.
- Anoxic brain damage such as cardiac arrest, exposure to manganese and carbon monoxide.
- Postencephalitic – as a result of encephalitis lethargica or Economo's disease.
- 1-methyl-4-phenyl-1,2,3,6-tetrahydropyridine toxicity – seen in drug abusers.

Also mention that atherosclerosis was previously thought to cause Parkinson's disease but this is no longer accepted as a causative factor.

Mention a few drugs which cause this syndrome.

Chlorpromazine, prochloperazine, metaclopramide.

What is the difference between rigidity and spasticity?

- Rigidity indicates increased tone affecting opposing muscle groups equally and is present throughout the range of passive movement. When smooth it is called 'lead pipe' rigidity and when intermittent it is termed 'cogwheel' rigidity. It is common in extrapyramidal syndromes.
- Spasticity of the clasp knife type is characterised by increased tone which is maximal at the beginning of movement and suddenly decreases as passive movement is continued. It chiefly occurs in the flexors of the upper limb and extensors of the lower limbs (anti-gravity muscles).

■ How would you manage a patient with Parkinson's syndrome?

  - If symptoms are mild, treat the patient with selegiline as it retards the progress of the degenerative disease.
  - If tremor is the main problem treat with anticholinergics such as benzhexol (contraindications are glaucoma or bladder symptoms).

- If bradykinesia is the main problem then treat with L-dopa with a decarboxylase inhibitor such as carbidopa or benserazide. Second line drugs are bromocriptine and amantadine.

Do you know of any substance which has been known to reverse Parkinson's disease in animals?

When monkeys were treated with G_{M1} ganglioside extracted from cow's brain the motor function was restored to nearly normal.

What are Parkinson plus syndromes?

Some patients have other neurological deficits in addition to Parkinson's syndrome. Examples of these so-called Parkinson plus syndromes are:

- Shy–Drager syndrome.
- Multiple system atrophy.
- Wilson's disease.
- Huntington's chorea.
- Cerebral palsy.

What is tardive dyskinesia?

Tardive dyskinesia is seen in patients on neuroleptics. Its manifestations are orofacial dyskinesia such as smacking and chewing lip movements, discrete dystonia, or choreiform movements and – rarely – rocking trunk movements. Withdrawing the offending drug will improve these symptoms over a period of 3–4 years, except in a small minority of patients.

James Parkinson (1755–1824) first reported six cases of this syndrome in 1817 (at the age of 62).
JC Steele, JC Richardson and J Olszewski were all US neurologists.
K von Economo (1876–1931) was an Austrian neurologist who also wrote on Wilson's disease.
GM Shy (1919–1967), a US neurologist, obtained his London MRCP in 1947.
GA Drager (1917–1967), US neurologist.
CD Marsden, contemporary Professor of Neurology, National Hospital, Queen's Square, London; his chief interest is Parkinson's disease and movement disorders.

References

Editorial (1990) Driving and Parkinson's disease. *Lancet* **336:** 781.
Lees, AJ (1986) L-Dopa treatment and Parkinson's disease. *Q J Med* **59:** 535.
Marsden, CD (1990) Parkinson's disease. *Lancet* **335:** 948–952.
Parkinson Study Group (1989) Effect of deprenyl (seligiline) on the progression of disability in early Parkinson's disease. *N Engl J Med* **321:** 1364.
Pearce, JMS (1990) Progression of Parkinson's disease. *Br Med J* **301:** 396.
Williams, A (1990) Cell implantation in Parkinson's disease. *Br Med J* **301:** 301.

| Case 38 | Cerebellar Syndrome |

Instruction

Examine this patient who presented with a history of falling to one side.
Demonstrate cerebellar signs.

Salient features

Perform the following examinations:

• Look for nystagmus: comment on the direction of the fast component.
• Tell the examiner you would like to ask the patient a few questions to assess his or her speech.
• Ask the patient to keep his or her arms outstretched; then give them a small push downward and look for rebound phenomenon.
• Examine for rapid alternating movements with the hand.
• Do the finger–nose test: look for past pointing and intention tremor.
• Do the heel–shin test.
• Examine the gait, in particular tandem walking.

• Tell the examiner you would like to examine the fundus for optic atrophy as demyelination is the commonest cause of cerebellar syndrome.

Questions

How may cerebellar signs manifest?

• Disorders of movement:
   Nystagmus.
   Scanning dysarthria
   Lack of finger–nose co-ordination (past pointing) – dysmetria.
   Rebound phenomenon – inability to arrest strong contraction on sudden removal of resistance.
   Intention tremor.
   Dysdiadochokinesis – impairment of rapid alternating movements (clumsy).

Dyssynergia – movements involving more than one joint are broken into parts.
- Hypotonia.
- Absent reflexes or pendular reflexes.
- Lack of co-ordination of gait – patient tends to fall towards the side of the lesion.

What are the causes of cerebellar syndrome?

- Demyelination (multiple sclerosis).
- Brain stem vascular lesion.
- Phenytoin toxicity.
- Alcoholic cerebellar degeneration.
- Space-occupying lesion in the posterior fossa including cerebellopontine angle tumour.
- Hypothyroidism (a reversible cause).
- Paraneoplastic manifestation of bronchogenic carcinoma.
- Friedreich's and other hereditary ataxias.
- Congenital malformations at the level of the foramen magnum.

How are cerebellar signs localised?

- Gait ataxia: anterior lobe.
- Truncal ataxia, titubation: flocculonodular lobe.
- Limb ataxia, especially upper limbs: lateral lobes.

If you are allowed to do one investigation which one would you choose in a patient with a suspected cerebellar lesion?

Magnetic resonance image (MRI) scan.

Case 39 | Jerky Nystagmus

Instruction

Examine this patient's eyes.
Test this patient's eye movements.

Salient features

* Horizontal nystagmus with fast components to right or left side (when eliciting nystagmus take care to keep your finger at least 2 feet away from the patient and avoid going laterally beyond the extent of binocular vision).
* Look for other cerebellar signs (see page 80).
* Tell the examiner that you would like to do the following:
  Examine the fundus for optic atrophy (multiple sclerosis).
  Take a history of vertigo (vestibular nystagmus).

Note. Remember that if the patient has vertical nystagmus in addition to horizontal nystagmus it is more likely to be vestibular nystagmus or brain stem disease.

Questions

What do you understand by the term 'nystagmus'?

Nystagmus is a series of involuntary, rhythmic oscillations of one or both eyes. It may be horizontal, vertical or rotatory.

What is pendular nystagmus?

In pendular nystagmus the oscillations are equal in speed and amplitude in both directions of movement. It may be seen on central gaze when the vision is poor, as in severe refractive error or macular disease.

What do you understand by the term 'jerky nystagmus'?

Jerky or phasic nystagmus is a condition in which eye movement in one direction is faster than that in the other. This is usually seen in the horizontal plane and is brought out by lateral gaze to one or both sides. It is seen with lesions of the cerebellum, vestibular apparatus or their connections in the brain stem.

What is dissociated nystagmus?

Dissociated or ataxic nystagmus is irregular nystagmus in the abducting eye. It is bilateral in multiple sclerosis, brain stem tumour and Wernicke's encephalopathy. It is unilateral in vascular disease of the brain stem. It is due to a lesion in the medial longitudinal fasciculus (which links the sixth nerve nucleus on one side to the medial rectus portion of the third nerve on the other side).

■ Where is the lesion in vestibular nystagmus?

It may be in one of two locations:

- Peripheral (labyrinth or vestibular nerve), as in labyrinthitis, Ménière's syndrome, acoustic neuroma, otitis media, head injury.
- Central (affecting vestibular nuclei), as in stroke, multiple sclerosis, tumours, alcoholism.

K Wernicke (1848–1904) graduated from Poland; although aware that a toxic factor was important in the aetiology he did not realise that this syndrome was due to a nutritional deficiency.
P Ménière (1799–1862), French ear, nose and throat specialist.

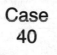

Case 40 Speech

Instruction

Ask this patient some questions.

Approach

- Ask the patient simple questions regarding personal details such as name, age, occupation, address and handedness (remember that over 90% of left-handed people have a dominant left hemisphere).
- Test the following:

- *Comprehension*
    Put your tongue out.
    Shut your eyes.
    Touch your nose.
    Smile.
    Two-step commands, such as touch your left ear with your right hand.
- *Orientation*
    Time–date.
    Place.

- *Name familiar objects*
    Pen.
    Coin.
    Watch.
- *Articulation*. Ask the patient to repeat the following:
    British constitution.
    West Register Street.
    Baby hippopotamus.
    Biblical criticism.
    Artillery.
- *Abbreviated mental test*
    Age.
    Address to recall: 42 West Street.
    Year.
    Time.
    Date of birth.
    Year of World War I or World War II.
    Name of this place.
    Recognition of two persons such as doctor, nurse.
    Name of the Monarch or Prime Minister.
    Count backwards from 20 to 1.
    Serially subtract 7 from 200.

Questions

What do you understand by the term 'dysphasia'?

Dysphasia is a disorder of the content of speech which usually follows a lesion of the dominant cortex:

- When the *speech defect* is expressive dysphasia or nominal dysphasia or motor dysphasia, the *site of lesion in the cortex* is the posterior inferior part of the dominant frontal lobe, i.e. *Broca's area.*
- When the *speech defect* is sensory dysphasia or receptive dysphasia, the *site of lesion in the cortex* is the superior temporal lobe or *Wernicke's area.*

What do you understand by the term 'dysarthria'?

Dysarthria is an inability to articulate properly due to the local lesions in the mouth or disorders of muscle speech or their connections. There is no disorder of content of speech. The causes of dysarthria are as follows:

- Stutter.
- Paralysis of cranial nerves – Bell's palsy, ninth, tenth and eleventh nerves.

- Cerebellar disease – staccato, scanning speech.
- Parkinson's speech – slow, quiet, slurred, monotonous.
- Pseudobulbar palsy – monotonous, high-pitched 'hot potato' speech.
- Progressive bulbar palsy – nasal.

What are the components of speech?

- Phonation: abnormality is called dysphonia.
- Articulation: abnormality is called dysarthria.
- Language: abnormality is called dysphasia.

What are the other dominant hemisphere functions?

- Right–left orientation.
- Finger identification.
- Calculation.

What are nondominant hemisphere functions?

- Drawing ability
- Topographic ability.
- Construction.
- Dressing.
- Facial recognition.
- Awareness of body and space.
- Motor persistence.

What are the parietal lobe signs?

- Loss of accurate localisation of touch, position, joint sense and temperature appreciation.
- Loss of two-point discrimination.
- Astereognosis.
- Dysgraphaesthesia
- Sensory inattention.
- Attention hemianopia, homonymous hemianopia or lower quadrantic hemianopia sometimes present.

Case 41	Expressive Dysphasia

Instruction

Ask this patient a few questions.

Salient features

- Patient has difficulty in finding the appropriate words, comprehension is intact and repetition may or may not be intact.
- Tell the examiner that you would like to carry out a neurological examination of the patient for a right-sided stroke.

Questions

Where is the lesion?

In the Broca's area which is located in the posterior portion of the third left frontal gyrus. It is the motor association cortex for face, tongue, lips and palate. It contains motor patterns necessary to produce speech.

How would you manage this patient?

- CT head scan to localise the affected area.
- Aspirin.
- Referral to the speech therapist.
- General rehabilitation of patient with stroke.

Pierre Paul Broca (1824–1880) was a Professor of Surgery in Paris. His notable achievements were in anthropology and his suggestion of cerebral localisation of speech was first made at the French Anthropological Society meeting in 1861. He is reported to have described muscular dystrophy (before Duchenne), venous spread of cancer (before Rokitansky) and rickets as a nutritional disorder (before Virchow).

References

Damasio, AR (1992) Medical progress: aphasia. *N Engl J Med* **326**: 531–539.
Geschwind, N (1971) Aphasia. *N Engl J Med* **284**: 654.

Case 42	Cerebellar Dysarthria

Instruction

Ask this patient a few questions.

Salient features

- The speech may be scanning (enunciation is difficult, words are produced slowly and in a measured fashion) or staccato (in bursts).
- Articulation is uneven, words are slurred and variations in pitch and loudness occur.

- Tell the examiner that you would like to carry out a neurological examination of the patient for cerebellar signs.
  See *Cerebellar Syndrome* (page 80) for discussion.

Questions

What do you understand by the term 'dysarthria'?

Dysarthria is impaired articulation of speech. It may result from lesions of muscles, myoneural junctions or motor neurons of lips, tongue, palate and pharynx. Common causes include mechanical defects such as ill fitting dentures or cleft palate. Dysarthria may also result from impaired hearing which begins in early childhood.

How would you test the different structures responsible for articulation?

- Lips: ask the patient to say, 'me, me, me'.
- Tongue: ask the patient to say, 'la, la, la'.
- Pharynx: ask the patient to say, 'kuh, gut'.
- Palate, larynx and expiratory muscles: ask the patient to say, 'ah'.

Articulation can also be tested by asking the patient to repeat the following:

- British constitution.
- Hippopotamus.
- Methodist Episcopal.
- Constantinople is the capital of Turkey.

| Case 43 | Third Cranial Nerve Palsy |

Instruction

Examine this patient's eyes.

Salient features

- Unilateral ptosis.
- Dilatation of the pupil.
- Squint due to the weakness of muscles supplied by the third nerve (superior, inferior, medial recti, inferior oblique). The eye will be in the position of abduction, i.e. down and out (if the fourth and sixth nerve are intact).

- Exclude associated fourth cranial nerve lesion (supplies the superior oblique) by tilting the head of the patient to the same side – the affected eye will intort if the fourth nerve is intact. Remember superior oblique intorts the eye (SIN).
- Tell the examiner that you would like to check the urine for sugar and the blood pressure.

Questions

What are the common causes of a third nerve palsy?

- Hypertension and diabetes are the most common causes of pupil-sparing third nerve palsy. (**Note.** the presence of pain is not a good discriminating feature between diabetes and aneurysm as pain is present in both.) Diabetic third nerve palsy usually recovers within 3 months.

- Multiple sclerosis.
- Aneurysms of posterior communicating artery (painful ophthalmoplegia).
- Trauma.
- Tumours, collagen vascular disorder, syphilis.
- Ophthalmoplegic migraine.
- Encephalitis.
- Parasellar neoplasms.
- Meningiomas at the wing of sphenoid.
- Basal meningitis.
- Carcinoma at the base of the skull.

How would you investigate such a patient?

- Blood pressure and urine for sugar.
- ESR to exclude temporal arteritis (in the elderly).
- Edrophonium (tensilon) test to exclude myasthenia if the pupil is not involved.
- Thyroid function tests and orbital ultrasound to exclude thyroid disease.
- CT scan of the head.
- Arteriography, especially when the pupil is involved and there is severe pain.

Do you know of any eponymous syndromes where the third cranial nerve is involved?

- Weber's syndrome, i.e. ipsilateral third nerve palsy with contralateral hemiplegia. The lesion is in the midbrain.
- Benedikt's syndrome, i.e. ipsilateral third nerve palsy with contralateral involuntary movements such as tremor, chorea and athetosis. It is due to a lesion of the red nucleus in the midbrain.

M Benedikt (1835–1920), an Austrian physician, described this syndrome in 1889.
Sir HD Weber (1823–1918) qualified in Bonn and worked at Guy's Hospital, London.

| Case 44 | Sixth Cranial Nerve Palsy |

Instruction

Examine this patient's eyes.

Salient features

- The eye is deviated medially and there is failure of lateral movement.
- The diplopia is maximal when looking towards the affected side. The two images are parallel and separated in the horizontal plane. The outer image comes from the affected eye and disappears when that eye is covered.
- Subtle weakness can be elicited by asking the patient to move his or her eyes in the direction of the affected muscle: the patient will have diplopia even though extraocular movements are full range.

- Tell the examiner that you would like to check the following:
    Blood pressure and urine sugar.
    Hearing and corneal sensation (early signs of acoustic neuroma).

Questions

What are the causes of sixth nerve palsy?

- Hypertension and diabetes.
- Raised intracranial pressure (false localising sign).
- Multiple sclerosis.
- Encephalitis.
- Acoustic neuroma, nasopharyngeal carcinoma.

Where is the nucleus of the sixth nerve located?

In the pons. (**Note.** The nuclei of the first four cranial nerves are situated above the pons and the nuclei of the last four cranial nerves are situated below the pons.)

■ Have you heard of Gradenigo's syndrome?

Inflammation of the tip of the temporal bone may involve the fifth and sixth cranial nerves as well as the greater superficial petrosal nerve, resulting in unilateral paralysis of the lateral rectus muscle, pain in the distribution of the trigeminal nerve (particularly its first division) and excessive lacrimation.

Do you know any eponymous syndromes where the pons is infarcted and consequently the sixth cranial nerve is involved?

- Millard–Gubler syndrome, in which there is ipsilateral sixth and seventh nerve palsy with contralateral hemiplegia.
- Foville's syndrome has all the features of Millard–Gubler with lateral conjugate gaze palsy.

What do you know about Tolosa–Hunt syndrome?

It is a syndrome characterised by unilateral recurrent pain in the retro-orbital region with palsy of the extraocular muscles due to involvement of the third, fourth, fifth and sixth cranial nerves. It has been attributed to inflammation of the cavernous sinus.

C Gradenigo (1859–1926), an Italian otolaryngologist, described this syndrome in 1904.
E Tolosa, Spanish neurosurgeon.
WE Hunt, American neurosurgeon.
ALJ Millard (1830–1915), French physician.
AM Gubler (1821–1915), Professor of Therapeutics in France.
ALF Foville (1799–1878), Professor of Physiology at Rouen, described his syndrome in 1848.

| Case 45 | Seventh Cranial Nerve Palsy – Lower Motor Neuron Type |

Instruction

Examine the cranial nerves.
Look at this patient's face.

Salient features

- Weakness of muscles of one half of the face – patient is unable to screw his or her eyes tightly shut or move the angle of the mouth on the affected side.

- Look at the external auditory meatus for herpes zoster (Ramsay Hunt syndrome)
- Look for parotid gland enlargement.
- Tell the examiner that you would like to do the following:
  Examine for taste (loss of taste in the involvement of chorda tympani).
  Check hearing for hyperacusis due to involvement of nerve to stapedius muscle.
  Examine the tympanic membrane for otitis media.

Questions

How would you differentiate between upper and lower motor neuron palsy?

In lower motor neuron palsy the whole half of the face on the affected side is involved. In upper motor neuron palsy the upper half of the face (the forehead) is spared.

What are the causes of bilateral nerve palsy?

- Guillain–Barré syndrome
- Sarcoidosis in the form of uveoparotid fever (Heerfordt's disease)
- Melkersson–Rosenthal syndrome, which is a triad of recurrent facial palsy, recurrent facial oedema and plication of the tongue.

Note. Myasthenia gravis may mimic bilateral facial nerve palsy.

What are causes of unilateral facial nerve palsy?

Lower motor neuron (all the muscles of one half of the face are affected):

- Bell's palsy (idiopathic).
- Herpes zoster.
- Old polio.
- Otitis media.
- Skull fracture.
- Cerebellopontine angle tumours.
- Parotid tumours.

Upper motor neuron (forehead spared):
- Stroke (hemiplegia).

Is the facial a motor nerve or a sensory nerve?

The facial nerve is predominantly a motor nerve and supplies all muscles concerned with facial expression and the stapedius muscle. Uncommonly, it may have a sensory component which is small – the nervus intermedius of Wrisberg. It conveys taste sensation from the anterior two thirds of the tongue and, probably, cutaneous impulses from the anterior wall of the external auditory canal.

How would you manage Bell's palsy?

- Physiotherapy: massage, electrical stimulation, splint to prevent drooping of the lower part of the face.
- Protection of the eye during sleep.
- A short course of dexamethasone 2 mg three times a day for 5 days and tapered over the next 5 days (should be given within 48 hours after onset).

How would you localise facial nerve palsy?

- Involvement of nuclei in the pons – associated ipsilateral sixth nerve palsy.
- Cerebellopontine angle lesion – associated fifth and eighth nerve involvement.
- Lesion in the bony canal – loss of taste (carried by lingual nerve) and hyperacusis (due to involvement of the nerve to stapedius).

■ Mention a few examples of facial synkinesis.

Facial synkinesis means that attempts to move one group of facial muscles result in contraction of associated muscles. It may be seen during anomalous regeneration of facial nerve. For example:

- If fibres originally connected with muscles of the face later innervate the lacrimal gland, anomalous secretion of tears (crocodile tears) may occur while eating.
- If fibres originally connected with the orbicularis oculi innervate the orbicularis oris, closure of the eyelids causes retraction of the mouth.
- Opening of the jaw may cause closure of the eyelids on the corresponding side (jaw-winking).

Have you heard of Möbius syndrome?

Congenital facial diplegia, congenital oculofacial paralysis and infantile nuclear aplasia. It consists of congenital bilateral facial palsy associated with third and sixth nerve palsies.

Sir Charles Bell (1774–1842) was Professor of Surgery in Edinburgh and a founder

member of the Middlesex Hospital in London. He discovered that the anterior and posterior spinal nerve roots were motor and sensory respectively.
James Ramsay Hunt (1874–1937), Professor of Neurology in New York.
PJ Möbius (1853–1907), German neurologist.

Case 46	Tremor

Instruction

Look at this patient's hands.
Demonstrate tremor.

Salient features

Patient 1:

- Coarse resting tremor which is slow (4–6 per second).
- Adduction–abduction of the thumb with flexion extension of fingers.
- The tremor is halted by purposive movements.

- Tell the examiner you would like to do the following:
    Look for cogwheel rigidity.
    Comment on mask-like facies.
    Check gait for festinatant gait.

  This patient has Parkinson's disease.

Patient 2: there is a 10-second physiological tremor which is brought on when the arms are outstretched. It can be amplified by laying a sheet of paper on the hands.

- Tell the examiner that you would like to do the following:
    Check for thyrotoxicosis.
    Take a history of alcoholism.
    Take a drug history (salbutamol, terbutaline).

Know whether tremor runs in the family (benign essential tremor).

Patient 3 does not have a resting tremor or a tremor with outstretched hands.

- Check for past pointing – the intention tremor of cerebellar disease.
- Tell the examiner that you would like to check for other cerebellar signs (see page 80).

Questions

What are tremors?

Involuntary movements which result from alternate contraction and relaxation of groups of muscles producing rhythmic oscillations about a joint or a group of joints.

How would you classify tremors?

- Resting tremor, as in Parkinson's disease.
- Postural tremor (brought on when the arms are outstretched) due to the following:
  Exaggerated physiological tremor, caused by anxiety, thyrotoxicosis, alcohol, drugs.
  Brain damage, seen in Wilson's disease, syphilis.
- Intention tremor (aggravated by voluntary movement) in cerebellar disease.

Mention a few involuntary movements.

- Chorea
- Athetosis.
- Hemiballismus.
- Fasciculation.
- Torticollis.
- Clonus.

References

Fahn, S (1972) Differential diagnosis of tremors. *Med Clin N Am* **56(6)**: 1363–1375.

Case 47   Peripheral Neuropathy

Instruction

Carry out a neurological examination of this patient's legs or arms.

Salient features

- Bilateral symmetrical sensory loss for all modalities with or without motor weakness.
- Look for evidence of the following:
- Diabetes mellitus (diabetic chart, insulin injection sites).
- Alcoholic liver disease.
- Vitamin B_{12} deficiency (anaemia, jaundice).
- Drugs.
- Chronic renal failure.
- Rheumatoid arthritis.
- Malignancy.
- Palpate for thickened nerves and look for signs of Charcot's joints.
- Tell the examiner that you would like to do the following:
    Check urine for sugar.
    Take a history of alcohol consumption and a drug history.

Questions

Mention a few causes of thickened nerves.

- Amyloidosis.
- Charcot–Marie–Tooth disease.
- Leprosy.
- Refsum's disease (retinitis pigmentosa, deafness and cerebellar damage).
- Déjérine–Sottas disease (hypertrophic peripheral neuropathy).

What are the causes of motor neuropathy?

- Guillain–Barré syndrome.
- Peroneal muscular atrophy.
- Lead toxicity.
- Porphyria.

What are the causes of mononeuritis multiplex?

- Diabetes mellitus.
- Polyarteritis nodosa.
- Rheumatoid arthritis.
- Wegener's granulomatosis.
- Sarcoidosis.
- Amyloidosis.
- SLE.
- Carcinomatosis.
- Churg–Strauss syndrome.

Mention a few causes for predominantly sensory neuropathy.

- Diabetes mellitus.
- Alcoholics.
- Deficiency of vitamins B_{12} and B_1.
- Chronic renal failure.
- Leprosy.

What are the types of neuropathy described in diabetes mellitus?

- Symmetrical mainly sensory polyneuropathy.
- Asymmetrical mainly motor polyneuropathy (diabetic amyotrophy).
- Mononeuropathy.
- Autonomic neuropathy.

What are the other effects of alcohol on the central nervous system?

- Wernicke's encephalopathy (ophthalmoplegia, nystagmus, confusion, neuropathy).
- Korsakoff's psychosis (recent memory loss and confabulation).
- Central pontine myelinolysis.
- Epilepsy.
- Myopathy.

K Wernicke (1848–1904) worked in Poland.
SS Korasakoff (1853–1900) Russian neuropsychiatrist.
J Churg (b. 1910) qualified in Poland and was Professor of Pathology in New York.
L Strauss, US pathologist, New York.

References

Harati, Y (1987) Diabetic peripheral neuropathies. *Ann Intern Med* **107**: 546.

Case 48	Charcot–Marie–Tooth Disease (Peroneal Muscular Atrophy)

Instruction

Examine this patient's legs.

Salient features

- Wasting of muscles of calves and thighs which stops abruptly, usually in the lower third of the thigh, and is described as 'stork' or 'spindle' legs, 'fat bottle' calves and 'inverted champagne bottles'.
- Pes cavus, clawing of toes.
- Weakness of dorsiflexion.
- Ankle jerks absent, plantars are downgoing or equivocal.
- Mild sensory impairment or no sensory loss.

- Feel for lateral popliteal nerve thickening (seen in some cases only).
- Look at the hands for small muscle wasting.
- Tell the examiner that you would like to know whether or not there is a family history of the disease.

Note. There are two distinctive clinical features of this disease. First, the muscular atrophy begins in distal portions of the affected muscles in the lower and upper limbs, unlike the global atrophy of motor neuron disease or muscular dystrophy. The atrophy then creeps upwards involving all the muscles. Second, the degree of disability is minimal in spite of the marked deformity.

Questions

What is the mode of inheritance?

Both autosomal dominant and recessive inheritances are seen in different families. In hereditary motor sensory neuropathy (HMSN) type I with dominant inheritance the locus is on the long arm of chromosome 1.

What are the three recognised forms?

- HMSN type I – a demyelinating neuropathy.
- HMSN type II – an axonal neuropathy.
- Distal spinal muscular atrophy.

What other uncommon features may these patients have?
Optic atrophy, retinitis pigmentosa, spastic paraparesis.

In which other condition is pes cavus seen?
Friedreich's ataxia.

What is the natural history of the disease?
The disease usually arrests in middle life.

How does the forme fruste of the disease manifest?
The form fruste may be seen in the family members of the Charcot–Marie–Tooth disease and it manifests as pes cavus and absent ankle jerks.

Mention a few conditions that Charcot is credited to have described for the first time.

• Ankle clonus.
• Tabes dorsalis and Charcot's joints.
• Multiple sclerosis.
• Peroneal muscular atrophy.
• Multiple cerebral aneurysms, called Charcot–Bouchard aneurysms.
• Hysteria.

The syndrome was originally described by JM Charcot (1825–1923) and P Marie (1853–1940) in 1886 at the Salpêtrière in Paris and independently by HH Tooth at St Bartholomew's Hospital and Queen's Square, London, at the same time.

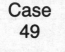

Case 49   Dystrophia Myotonica

Instruction

Look at this patient's face.
Examine this patient's cranial nerve.

Salient features

- While shaking hands with the patient note the myotonia.
- Mention the following features:

- Frontal baldness. (**Note.** The patient may be wearing a wig and it is important to mention that the patient is wearing one.)
- Ptosis (bilateral or unilateral) with a *smooth* forehead.
- Cataracts or evidence of surgery for cataracts.
- Difficulty in opening the eyes after firm closure.
- Expressionless face ('hatchet face') with wasting of temporalis, masseters and *sternomastoid*.

- Test:
  Sternomastoids.
  Distal muscles of the upper limbs for wasting, percussion myotonia over thenar muscles, and weakness.
- Tell the examiner that you would like to do the following:
  Ask the patient whether or not he (or she) has dysphagia (oesophageal involvement).
  Check the urine for sugar (diabetes mellitus).
  Test higher intellectual function (low IQ).
  Examine for gynaecomastia and testicular atrophy.

Questions

What is the inheritance of this condition?

Autosomal dominant and the gene is located on chromosome 19. It usually presents in the third and fourth decades. The disease tends to be worse in successive generations.

What are other features of this condition?

- Cardiomyopathy and cardiac conduction defects.
- Respiratory infection (low serum immunoglobulin IgG).
- Somnolence.
- External ophthalmoplegia (occasionally).

What do you understand by myotonia?

It is the continued contraction of the muscle after voluntary contraction ceases, followed by impaired relaxation.

What therapeutic modalities are available?

Procainamide or phenytoin have been used in *disabling* myotonia. No treatment has altered the course of progressive weakness.

What other form of myotonia do you know?

Myotonia congenita, which is an autosomal dominant condition and presents at birth with feeding difficulties. The myotonia improves with age and there is no dystrophy.

If this patient requires major surgery, what fact would you keep in mind?

Patients with dystrophia myotonica tend to do poorly after the administration of general anaesthetic (due to impaired cardiorespiratory malfunction) and will require intensive postoperative observation.

Mention some causes of bilateral ptosis?

- Myasthenia gravis.
- Congenital muscular dystrophies.
- Ocular myopathy.
- Syphilis.

What is the pathognomonic pattern of cataract in dystrophia myotonica?

Stellate cataract.

The patient's sister is worried about risks to her offspring. What tests would you do?

- Clinical examination.
- Electromyogram (EMG).
- Slit lamp examination for cataracts.

Is prenatal diagnosis available?

Yes – in some families. The myotonic dystrophy gene is linked to the ABH secretor gene. However, not all families are informative.

What is the characteristic EMG finding?

Waxing and waning of the potentials, known as the dive bomber effect.

Professor Kay Davies, Director of Research, Hammersmith Hospital, whose chief interest is genetics.

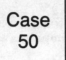

Proximal Myopathy

Instruction

Perform a neurological examination of this patient's arms or legs.

Salient features

- Weakness of proximal muscles.
- Patient has difficulty in standing from the sitting position (getting up from chairs, getting off the commode) or difficulty in combing his or her hair.

- Check the gait, looking for a waddling gait.
- Look for an underlying cause:
    Diabetic amyotrophy (asymmetrical, usually in the lower limbs in non-insulin-dependent diabetes mellitus).
    Cushing's syndrome (history of steroid ingestion).
    Thyrotoxicosis (look for eye signs, goitre, rapid pulse, tremor).
    Polymyositis (heliotropic rash, tender muscles).
    Carcinomatous neuropathy.
    Osteomalacia.
    Hereditary muscular dystrophy.

Questions

What is Gowers' sign?

In severe proximal myopathy of the lower limbs the patient on rising from the floor uses his or her hands to climb up him- or herself. It has been classically described in Duchenne muscular dystrophy.

What do you know about diabetic amyotrophy?

It is an asymmetrical motor polyneuropathy which presents with asymmetrical weakness and wasting of the proximal muscles of the lower limbs and sometimes upper limbs. It is usually accompanied by severe pain. The prognosis is good and most patients recover over months or years with good diabetic control.

Sir WR Gowers (1845–1915), Professor of Medicine at University College Hospital, London, invented a haemoglobinometer, personally illustrated an atlas of ophthalmology, wrote a book on spinal cord diseases and a manual on the nervous system. He also founded a society of medical stenographers.

Case 51	Deformity of a Lower Limb

Instruction

Examine the lower limbs of this patient who has had this abnormality since childhood.

Salient features

- Wasting and deformity of one lower limb (or both with one side being more than the other).
- Fasciculations.
- Normal tone in both lower limbs.

- Check sensory system.
- Examine the lower spine for tuft of hair (spina bifida).

Note. Always check the gait and test for Romberg's sign.

- Tell the examiner that you would like to ask the patient about the following:
    Bladder symptoms.
    History of trauma.

Questions

What is your differential diagnosis?

- Old poliomyelitis.
- Spina bifida.

What are the causes of lower motor neuron signs in the legs?

● Peripheral neuropathy.
● Prolapsed intervertebral disc.
● Diabetic amyotrophy.
● Poliomyelitis.
● Cauda equina lesions.
● Motor neuron disease.

MH Romberg (1795–1873), German neurologist and Professor of Medicine in Berlin.

Case 52   Multiple Sclerosis

Instruction

Examine this patient's eyes (*patient 1*).

Salient features

● Optic atrophy.
● Nystagmus.
● Internuclear ophthalmoplegia.

● Tell the examiner that you would like to look for features for cerebellar syndrome and do a full neurological examination.

Instruction

Examine this patient's legs (*patient 2*).

Salient features

- Spastic paraparesis (increased tone, upgoing plantars, weakness, brisk reflexes and ankle or patellar clonus).
- Impaired co-ordination on heel–shin test (if there is marked weakness then this test may be unreliable).

- Check abdominal reflexes.
- Tell the examiner that you would like to do the following:
  Take a history of sphincter incontinence, particularly of the bladder.
  Look for optic atrophy and cerebellar signs.

In such patients remember that spinal cord compression should be ruled out before making a diagnosis of multiple sclerosis.

Some examiners may consider it insensitive to use the term 'multiple sclerosis' in front of the patient and may prefer that the candidate uses the term 'demyelinating disorder' instead.

Questions

What investigations would you consider?

- Spinal X-rays, including both cervical and thoracic regions.
- Lumbar puncture: total protein may be elevated (in 60% of cases) with increase in IgG (in 40%) and oligoclonal bands (in 80%) on electrophoresis.
- Visual evoked potentials: despite normal visual function there may be prolonged latency in cortical response to a pattern stimulus. This indicates a delay in conduction in the visual pathways.
- MRI scan of the brain: about 50% of patients with early multiple sclerosis in the spinal cord show abnormal areas in the periventricular white matter.
- Serum B_{12} – to exclude subacute degeneration of the cord.

Mention a few causes of bilateral pyramidal lesions affecting the lower limbs?

- Cord compression.
- Multiple sclerosis.
- Cervical spondylosis.
- Transverse myelitis.
- Motor neuron disease.
- Vitamin B_{12} deficiency.
- Cerebrovascular disease.

What are the main ways in which multiple sclerosis can present?

- Optic neuritis (in 40% of cases), resulting in partial loss of vision.
- Weakness of one or more limbs.
- Tingling in the extremities due to posterior column involvement.
- Diplopia.
- Nystagmus, cerebellar ataxia.
- Vertigo.

What is the natural history of multiple sclerosis?

The course of the disease is extremely variable. The onset may be acute, subacute or insidious. The course may be rapidly downhill, or may spontaneously remit for periods lasting from days to years before a second exacerbation.

■ What is Lhermitte's sign?

A tingling or electric-shock-like sensation which radiates to the arms, down the back or into the legs on flexion of the patient's neck. It has also been called the barber's chair sign.

What is Uhthoff's symptom?

The exacerbation of symptoms of multiple sclerosis during a hot bath.

Do you know of any criteria for diagnosis of multiple sclerosis?

Poser's criteria: a history of two episodes of neurological deficit and objective clinical signs of lesions at more than one site within the central nervous system (CNS) establishes a diagnosis of definite multiple sclerosis. In the presence of only one clinical sign the demonstration of an additional lesion by laboratory tests – such as evoked potentials, MRI, CT, or urological studies – also fulfils the criteria.

A diagnosis of probable multiple sclerosis is defined as either two attacks with clinical evidence of one lesion or one attack with clinical evidence of two lesions.

Which conditions may be considered forme fruste of multiple sclerosis?

- Optic neuritis.
- Single episode of transverse myelitis with optic neuritis.

Does pregnancy affect the clinical features of multiple sclerosis?

Pregnancy itself may have a mildly protective effect but there is an increased risk of relapse during puerperium; overall, the effect on the course of the disease is probably negligible.

What is the role of exercise in the treatment of such patients?

Patients should be encouraged to keep active during remission and to avoid excessive physical exercise during relapses.

JL Lhermitte (1877–1959), a French neurologist and neuropsychiatrist, wrote extensively on spinal injuries, myoclonus, internuclear ophthalmoplegia and chorea.

References

McDonald, WI (1992) Multiple sclerosis: diagnostic optimism. *Br Med J* **304**: 1259.
Webb, HE (1992) Multiple sclerosis: therapeutic pessimism. *Br Med J* **305**: 1260.

Case 53	Abnormal Gait

Instruction

Look at this patient while he or she walks.
Test this patient's gait.

Salient features

Cerebellar gait: the patient has a broad based gait, reeling and lurching to one side.
- Tell the examiner that you would like to examine for other cerebellar signs (see page 80).

Parkinsonian gait: the steps are small and shuffling, and the patient walks in a haste (festinates). The entire body stoops forwards and the feet must hurry to keep up with it as if trying to catch up with a centre of gravity. There is associated loss of arm swing and mask-like facies.
- Tell the examiner that you would like to look for other signs of Parkinson's syndrome (see page 77).

Hemiplegic gait: the gait is slow, spastic and shuffling. The affected leg is circumducted, rotated in a semicircle with each step. The upper limb is flexed and the lower limb extended.

Sensory ataxia gait: the feet stamp, the movement of the legs bearing no relation to the position of the legs in space since proprioception is impaired or absent. The patient has to look down at the ground in order to compensate for the loss of proprioception.
- Check for Romberg's sign, vibration and position sense.
- Sensory ataxia gait may be due to the following:
    Tabes dorsalis.
    Subacute combined degeneration of the cord.
- Tell the examiner that you would like to look for Argyll Robertson pupils and anaemia.

High steppage gait is usually unilateral and is due to foot drop. The patient has to lift the foot high in order to avoid dragging the forefoot.
- It may be due to the following:
    Lateral popliteal nerve palsy.
    Poliomyelitis, Charcot–Marie–Tooth disease.
    Lead or arsenic poisoning.

Scissor gait is seen in spastic paraplegia.
- Tell the examiner that the underlying aetiology would probably be cord compression or multiple sclerosis.

Waddling gait is seen in proximal muscle weakness (Cushing's syndrome, osteomalacia, thyrotoxicosis, polymyositis, diabetes, hereditary muscular dystrophies).

| Case 54 | Wasting of the Small Muscles of the Hand |

Instruction

Examine this patient's hands.
Ask the patient if his or her hands are painful.

Salient features

- Wasting of thenar and hypothenar eminences and dorsal interossei.
- Look for joint deformity and swelling.
- Look for fasciculations.
- Check sensation over index and little fingers.
- Test grip and pincer movements.
- Test for median and ulnar nerve compression.
- Ask the patient to unbutton the clothes or to write.
- Palpate for cervical ribs.
- Look for Horner's syndrome.
- Examine the neck and test neck movements.

Remember that the causes of bilateral wasted hands are as follows:

- Rheumatoid arthritis.
- Old age.
- Cervical spondylosis.
- Bilateral cervical ribs.
- Motor neuron disease.
- Syringomyelia.
- Charcot–Marie–Tooth disease.
- Guillain–Barré syndrome.
- Bilateral median and ulnar nerve lesions.

If the wasting is seen in one hand only then in addition to the above causes consider the following:

- Brachial plexus trauma.
- Pancoast's tumour.
- Cervical cord lesions.
- Malignant infiltration of the brachial plexus.

Questions

At what level is the lesion?

C8, T1.

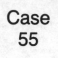

Case 55   Dermatomyositis

Instruction

Examine this patient.

Salient features

- Heliotrope rash or purplish blue rash around the eyes, back of the hands, knuckles (Gottron's sign) and around the finger nails.
- Proximal muscle weakness and tenderness of muscles.
- Neck flexor weakness in two thirds of cases.

- Tell the examiner that you would like to take a history of the following:
    Dysphagia.
    Dysphonia.
- If the patient is more than 40 years old, tell the examiner that you would like to look for an underlying neoplasm.

Questions

What investigations would you like to do?

- Serum creatine phosphokinase (CPK) levels (mirrors disease activity).
- EMG.
- Muscle biopsy.

How would you treat such patients?

- Most patients respond to steroids: prednisone is the first line drug for the empirical treatment of polymyositis and dermatomyositis.
- Resistant cases may benefit from methotrexate and azathioprine.
- Those with an underlying neoplasm may remit following treatment of the tumour.

What are the EMG findings in an affected muscle?

Spontaneous fibrillation, salvos of repetitive potentials and short duration of polyphasic potentials of low amplitude.

What features will a muscle biopsy show?

Necrosis and phagocytosis of muscle fibres, and interstitial and perivascular infiltration of inflammatory cells.

How would you classify polymyositis–dermatomyositis?

Classification of Bohan et al is as follows:
Group I, primary idiopathic polymyositis.
Group II, primary idiopathic dermatomyositis.
Group III, dermatomyositis (or polymyositis) associated with neoplasia.
Group IV, childhood dermatomyositis (or polymyositis) associated with vasculitis.
Group V, polymyositis (or dermatomyositis) with associated collagen vascular disease.

Mention a few disorders associated with myositis.

Sarcoid myositis, focal nodular myositis, infectious polymyositis (Lyme disease, toxoplasma), inclusion body myositis, eosinophilic myositis.

H Gottron, German dermatologist.

References

Bohan, A, Peter, JB, Bowman, R., Pearson CM et al (1977) A computer-assisted analysis of 153 patients with polymyositis and dermatomyositis. *Medicine* **56**: 255.

Dalakas, MC (1991) Medical progress: polymyositis, dermatomyositis, and inclusion-body myositis. *N Engl J Med* **325**: 1487.

Lakhanpal, S, Bunch, TW, Ilstrup, DM, Melton, LJ III et al (1986) Polymyositis–dermatomyositis and malignant lesions. Does an association exist? *Mayo Clin Proc* **61**: 645.

Case 56	Facioscapulohumeral Dystrophy (Landouzy–Déjérine Syndrome)

Instruction

Perform a neurological examination of this patient's cranial nerves and upper limbs.

Salient features

In the face:

- Prominent ptosis.
- Difficulty in closing the eyes.
- Marked facial weakness, resulting in a dull, expressionless face with lips open and slack, and inability to whistle, puff the cheeks or smile.
- Speech is impaired due to difficulty in articulation of labial consonants.

In the neck:

- Wasted sternomastoids and marked weakness of neck muscles.

Shoulder girdle:

- Winging of scapula.
- Lower pectorals and lower trapezii severely affected.
- Weakness of triceps and biceps.
- True hypertrophy of deltoids to compensate for other muscles.
- Absent biceps and triceps jerk.

Uncommon features: congenital absence of pectoralis, biceps or brachioradialis; tibialis anterior may be the only muscle involved outside the shoulder girdle.

Questions

What is the mode of inheritance?

Autosomal dominant, both sexes equally affected.

Are higher mental functions affected in this condition?

The IQ is normal in such patients.

What is the life span in such a patient?

Normal.

What is the age of onset of this disorder?

Between 10 and 40 years.

Are muscle enzymes raised in this condition?

No; the enzyme levels remain normal.

LTJ Landouzy (1845–1917), Professor of Therapeutics in Paris; although better remembered for the description of the syndrome which bears his name, his major research interest was tuberculosis.
JJ Déjérine (1849–1917), a French neurologist, was a pioneer in the localisation of function in the brain.

| Case 57 | Limb Girdle Dystrophy |

Instruction

Perform a neurological examination of this patient's upper and lower limbs.

Salient features

Upper limbs:

- Biceps and brachioradialis are involved late; wrist extensors are first involved when it extends into the wrist.
- Deltoids may show pseudohypertrophy and are spared until late.

Lower limbs:

- In the early stages of the disease, hip flexors and glutei are weak.
- There is early wasting of medial quadriceps and tibialis anterior.
- Lateral quadriceps and calves may show hypertrophy.

Note. The face is never affected.

Questions

What is the mode of inheritance?

Autosomal recessive, males and females equally affected.

What is the age of onset?

Between 10 and 30 years, causing disability 10–20 years after onset.

How is the intelligence affected?

It is unaffected and IQ is normal.

Is the life span affected?

No.

What happens to the serum enzymes?

The serum enzymes are slightly affected or normal.

Sir Roger Bannister, contemporary Neurologist, Oxford whose main interest is autonomic failure. He is the first person to run the four minute mile.
Lord Walton, contemporary Professor of Neurology, Oxford and Newcastle whose main interest is muscular diseases.

| Case 58 | Myasthenia Gravis |

Instruction

This patient complains of drooping of the eyelids in the evenings; examine this patient.

Salient features

- The patient may have obvious ptosis.
- Remember that *fatigability* is the hallmark of myasthenia gravis.
- Check for worsening of ptosis on sustained upward gaze.
- Check extraocular movements for diplopia and variable squint.
- Comment on snarling face when the patient attempts to smile.
- Tell the examiner that you would like to know whether or not the weakness is more marked in the evening.
- Tell the examiner that myasthenia is associated with thyrotoxicosis, diabetes mellitus, rheumatoid arthritis, SLE, thymoma.

Questions

What groups of muscles are commonly involved?

Muscles affected are as follows, in order of likelihood: extraocular, bulbar, neck, limb girdle, distal limbs, trunk.

What investigations would you like to do in this patient?

- Edrophonium (Tensilon) test.
- Vital capacity.
- X-ray of mediastinum.
- CT scan of the chest.
- Acetylcholine receptor antibodies (present in more than 80% of cases).
- Plasma thyroxine (to rule out an associated thyroid disorder).
- Antistriated muscle antibody (seen in association with thymoma).
- EMG (abnormalities include a decremental response to tetanic train stimulation at 5–10 Hz, and evidence of neuromuscular blockade is seen on single-fibre EMG in the form of jitter and blocking of motor action potentials).

What is the differential diagnosis?

- Botulism.
- Eaton–Lambert syndrome.

What are the treatment modalities available?

- Symptomatic treatment entails administration of an anticholinesterase, e.g. pyridostigmine, given up to five times per day.
- Definitive treatment entails immunosuppression, e.g. steroids, azathioprine, cyclosporin, plasmapheresis, thymectomy.

If this patient develops an infection which group of antibiotics would you avoid?

Aminoglycosides.

Mention a few exacerbating features.

Fatigue, exercise, infection, emotion, change of climate, pregnancy, magnesium enemas, drugs (aminoglycosides, propranolol, morphine, barbiturates, procainamide, quinidine).

What do you know about Eaton–Lambert syndrome?

Eaton–Lambert syndrome is a myasthenic disorder associated with malignancy. The pelvic girdle and thighs are almost invariably involved. EMG is diagnostic. In the rested muscle there is a marked depression of neuromuscular transmission after a single submaximal stimulus and a marked facilitation of response during repetitive stimulation at rates greater than 10 per second.

What is myasthenic crisis?

Exacerbation of myasthenia. The need for artificial ventilation occurs in about 10% of patients with myasthenia. Those with bulbar and respiratory infection are prone to respiratory infection. The crisis can be precipitated by respiratory infection and surgery. Such patients should be closely monitored for pulmonary function. Those on artificial ventilation are not given anticholinergics as this avoids stimulation of pulmonary secretions and uncertainties about overdosage.

How does a cholinergic crisis manifest?

Excessive salivation, confusion, lacrimation, miosis, pallor and collapse. It is important to avoid edrophonium in such patients.

Mention a few associated disorders.

Thyroid disorders (thyrotoxicosis, hypothyroidism), rheumatoid arthritis, diabetes mellitus, dermatomyositis, pernicious anaemia, SLE, Sjögren's disease, sarcoidosis and pemphigus.

What is the role of thymectomy in such patients?

In the case of a thymoma, a thymectomy is necessary to prevent tumour spread although most thymomas are benign. In the absence of a tumour, thymectomy has been found to be beneficial in 85% of patients and 35% go into drug-free remission. The improvement is noticed 1–10 years after surgery. The role of thymectomy in ocular myasthenia, in adults over 55 years of age and in children is still under debate.

LM Eaton (1905–1958), Professor of Neurology, Mayo Clinic, Rochester, Minnesota.
EH Lambert (b. 1915), Professor of Physiology, University of Minnesota.
Sir Samuel Wilks (1824–1911), physician, Guy's Hospital, London. Myasthenia gravis was known as Wilks' syndrome.

References

Fonseca, V, Harvard, CWH (1990) The natural course of myasthenia gravis. *Br Med J* **300**: 1409,
Lambert, EH & Eaton, LM (1957) Electromyography and electric stimulation of nerves in diseases of the motor unit. *JAMA* **163**: 1117.
O'Neill, JH, Murray, NM, Newsom-Davies J (1988) The Eaton–Lambert syndrome. *Brain* **111**: 577 (a review of 50 cases).
Seybold, ME (1983) Myasthenia gravis. A clinical and basic science review. *JAMA* **250**: 2516.

Case 59 | Thomsen's Disease (Myotonia Congenita)

Instruction

Look at this patient.

Salient features

- Diffuse muscle hypertrophy.
- Myotonia – may be apparent while shaking hands with the people.

- Tell the examiner that you would like to do the following:
    Ask the patient whether or not there is any seasonal variation in symptoms – myotonia is worse in winter due to the cold.
    Take a family history – inheritance is autosomal dominant.

Questions

How is the disease recognised in infancy?

Myotonia is present from birth and may be recognised by the child's peculiar cry. Also noticed in early infancy are difficulty in feeding and inability to reopen the eyes while having the face washed.

When does muscle hypertrophy manifest?

It is usually apparent in the second decade.

What is the cause of muscle hypertrophy?

It is due to almost continual involuntary isometric exercise.

What is the life expectancy in such patients?

These patients have a normal life expectancy.

What drugs would you use to ameliorate the myotonia?

Procainamide, quinidine.

In which other conditions is myotonia seen?

- Myotonia dystrophica.
- Paramyotonia congenita (episodic myotonia after exposure to the cold).
- Drugs such as clofibrate.

AJT Thomsen (1815–1896) was a Danish physician who described this condition in his family and himself in 1876.

Case 60 | Friedreich's Ataxia

Instruction

Perform a neurological examination of this patient's legs.

Salient features

- Pes cavus.
- Pyramidal weakness in the legs.
- Cerebellar signs, ataxia being a constant sign.
- Impaired vibration and joint sense.
- Absent ankle jerks with upgoing plantars.

- Tell the examiner that you would like to do the following investigations:
    Check for nystagmus (present in 25% of cases), scanning speech, intention tremor.
    Examine the heart for hypertrophic cardiomyopathy.
    Check the eyes for optic atrophy (present in 30% of cases).
    Check the spine for kyphoscoliosis.
    Check urine for sugar (10% of patients have diabetes).
    Check IQ, looking for intellectual deterioration.

Questions

What is the mode of inheritance?

Autosomal recessive or, rarely, sex linked.

What is the age of onset?

Between 6 to 18 years of age.

Why are the deep tendon reflexes absent even though plantars are upgoing?

This is due to a combination of pyramidal weakness with peripheral neuropathy.

In which other condition is there a mixture of cerebellar, pyramidal and dorsal column signs?

Multiple sclerosis.

Mention a few conditions with absent knee jerks and upgoing plantars.

- Peripheral neuropathy in a stroke patient.
- Motor neuron disease.
- Conus medullaris – cauda lesion.
- Tabes dorsalis.
- Subacute combined degeneration of the spinal cord.

What is the forme fruste of this condition?

Pes cavus or hammer toes, without any other signs, are seen in family members of such patients.

On which chromosome is the gene for this disorder localised?

Chromosome 9.

What are the clinical criteria for diagnosis of Friedreich's ataxia?

Harding's criteria:

- Essential criteria are onset before the age of 25 years, ataxia of limbs and gait, absent knee and ankle jerks, extensor plantars, motor conduction velocity greater than $40\,\mathrm{m\,s^{-1}}$, small or absent sensory nerve action potentials, dysarthria within 5 years of onset.
- Additional criteria (present in two thirds) are scoliosis, pyramidal weakness of lower limbs, absent upper limb reflexes, joint position and vibration loss in legs, abnormal ECG, pes cavus.

- Other features (present in less than 50% of cases) are nystagmus, optic atrophy, deafness, distal wasting and diabetes.

Name a few eponymous syndromes with cerebellar degeneration.

- Roussy–Lévy disease: hereditary spinocerebellar degeneration with atrophy of lower limb muscles and loss of deep tendon reflexes.
- Refsum's disease (see page 373).
- Bassen–Kornzweig syndrome (see page 373).

Nikolaus Friedreich (1825–1882), Professor of Pathology and neurologist in Heidelberg, described this condition, in a series of papers from 1861 to 1876.
Anita Harding, contemporary Professor of Neurology at National Hospital, Queens Square, London.
G Roussy (1874–1948), French neuropathologist.
G Levy (b. 1881), French neurologist.
S Refsum, Norwegian physician.

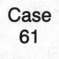

| Case 61 | Motor Neuron Disease |

Instruction

Examine this patient's cranial nerves.
Examine this patient's upper limbs.
Examine this patient's lower limbs.

Salient features

- Fasciculations, absent reflexes and weakness in the upper limbs.
- Spasticity, exaggerated reflexes and upgoing plantars in lower limbs.
- Sluggish palatal movements, absent gag reflex, brisk jaw jerk.

A combination of the above signs may be seen.

Questions

What important cause should be ruled out before making a firm diagnosis of motor neuron disease?

A cord compression may cause a similar clinical picture and hence it is important to do a myelogram to exclude it.

What are the characteristic features of this disease?

- It rarely begins before the age of 40.
- Sensory symptoms or signs are not seen.
- Sphincters are always spared.
- The disease is fatal within 5 to 7 years.

What are the clinical patterns of motor neuron disease?

- Bulbar: bulbar or pseudobulbar palsy (25% of cases).
- Amyotrophic lateral sclerosis (50% of cases): flaccid arms and spastic legs.
- Progressive muscular atrophy (25% of cases): a lesion in the anterior horn cells affecting the distal muscles.
- Primary lateral sclerosis (rare): signs progress from an upper motor neuron pattern to a lower motor neuron type.

What is the pathology of motor neuron disease?

Its clinical manifestations are a result of degeneration of Betz cells, pyramidal tracts, cranial nerve nuclei and anterior horn cells. Both upper and lower motor neurons may be involved but sensory involvement is not seen.

What do you know about the heredity of amyotrophic lateral sclerosis?

Most cases are sporadic. Five to ten per cent of cases are familial, and familial amyotrophic lateral sclerosis is linked to a gene on the long arm of chromosome 21.

References

Mitsumoto, H, Hanson, MR & Chad, DA (1988) Amyotrophic lateral sclerosis. Recent advances in pathogenesis and therapeutic trials. *Arch Neurol* 45: 189.
Siddique, T, Figlewicz, DA, Periak-Vance MA et al (1991) Linkage of a gene causing familial amyotrophic lateral sclerosis to chromosome 21 and evidence of genetic locus heterogeneity. *N Engl J Med* 324: 1381.

<table>
<tr><td>Case
62</td><td>Neurofibromatosis</td></tr>
</table>

Instruction

Examine this patient.

Salient features

- Multiple neurofibroma and café-au-lait spots.

Examine the following:
- The axilla for freckles.
- Visual acuity and fundus for optic glioma.
- Hearing and corneal sensation for acoustic neuroma.
- The iris for Lisch nodules (often apparent only by slit lamp examination).
- The spine for kyphoscoliosis.
- Tell the examiner that you would like to check the blood pressure (for phaeochromocytoma).

Questions

What are the criteria for neurofibromatosis type 1 (Recklinghausen's disease)?

Neurofibromatosis type 1 may be diagnosed when two or more of the following are present:

- Six or more café-au-lait spots, the greatest diameter of which is more than 5 mm in prepubertal patients and more than 15 mm in postpubertal patients.
- Two or more neurofibromas or one plexiform neurofibroma.
- Freckling in the axilla or inguinal region.
- Optic glioma.
- Two or more Lisch nodules (iris hamartoma).
- A distinctive osseous lesion such as sphenoid dysplasia or thinning of long bone cortex with or without pseudoarthroses.
- A parent, sibling or child with neurofibromatosis according to the above criteria.

What are the criteria for neurofibromatosis type 2?

- Bilateral eighth nerve palsy confirmed by either CT or MRI.
- A parent, sibling or child with neurofibromatosis type 2 and either unilateral eighth nerve mass or any two of the following: neurofibroma, meningioma, glioma, schwannoma or juvenile posterior subcapsular lenticular opacity.

What is the significance of the Lisch nodules?

Lisch nodules are melanocytic hamartomas that appear as well-defined, dome-shaped elevations projecting from the surface of the iris and are clear to yellow and brown. They are an important tool in establishing the diagnosis of neurofibromatosis 1 and providing accurate genetic counselling.

What do you know about the inheritance of these two disorders?

Both are autosomal dominant syndromes, type 1 being carried on chromosome 17 and type 2 being carried on chromosome 22.

Friedreich Daniel von Recklinghausen (1833–1910) was Professor of Pathology successively at Könisberg, Würzburg and Strasbourg. He also described another disease – arthritis deformans neoplastica – to which his name is attached.

References

Barker, D, Wright, E, Nquyen, K et al (1987) Gene for von Recklinghausen's neurofibromatosis is in the pericentric region of chromosome 17. *Science* **236**: 110.

Lubs, ME, Bauer, MS, Formas, ME & Djokic, B (1991) Lisch nodules in neurofibromatosis type 1. *N Engl J Med* **324**: 1264.

Martuza, RL & Eldridge, R (1988) Neurofibromatosis 2. *N Engl J Med* **318**: 685.

Riccardi, VM (1991) Neurofibromatosis: past, present and future. *N Engl J Med* **324**: 1283.

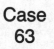

Case 63   Syringomyelia

Instruction

Examine this patient's arms.

Salient features

- Wasting and weakness of the small muscles of the hands and forearm (if fasciculation is seen then the other diagnosis that comes to mind at this stage is motor neuron disease).
- Tone and deep tendon reflexes are diminished.
- Loss of pain and temperature sensation with intact vibration, light touch and joint position sense. Note that this will be the underlying cause for any burns present. There may be Charcot's joints of the shoulder and elbow.
- Examine vibration sense over the fingers, lower end of radius, elbow and clavicles (note that vibration sense is impaired only at a late stage).

- Look for Horner's syndrome.
- Examine the neck posteriorly for scar of previous surgery.
- Ask if you may examine the following:
  The lower limbs for pyramidal signs.
  The face for loss of temperature and pain sensation (starting from the outer part of the face and progressing forward, looking for the 'onion skin pattern' of sensory loss due to a lesion in the spinal nucleus of the fifth cranial nerve which extends from the pons down to the upper cervical cord).
  For lower cranial nerve palsy.
  For nystagmus and ataxia (due to involvement of the medial longitudinal bundle from C5 upwards).
  For kyphoscoliosis (due to paravertebral muscle involvement).

Questions

What is *la main succulente*?

In some patients with syringomyelia the hands will have an ugly appearance due to trophic and vasomotor disturbances;

these commonly result in cold, cyanosed and swollen fingers and palms.

What investigations would you do?

MRI scan – in the past, myelograms were done to confirm the diagnosis but these were associated with deterioration of the condition in a large number of patients.

What associated abnormalities may be present?

Arnold–Chiari malformation, spina bifida, bony defects around the foramen magnum, hydrocephalus, spinal cord tumours.

What conditions may present with a similar picture?

Intramedullary tumours of the spinal cord, haematomyelia, craniovertebral anomalies and late sequelae of spinal cord injuries.

What treatment is available?

Syringoperitoneal shunting.

What other causes of Charcot's joints do you know?

- Diabetes mellitus, especially when toes and ankles are affected.
- Tabes dorsalis, especially when knee and hip joints are affected.

The term 'syringomyelia' (from *syrinx*, a pipe or tube) was first used by Ollivier in 1824, in his monograph on diseases of the spinal cord, to denote cavity formation. It denotes the presence of a large, fluid-filled cavity in the grey matter of the spinal cord which is in communication with the central canal and contains CSF.
J Arnold (1835–1915), Professor of Pathology at Heidelberg.
H Chiari (1851–1916), Austrian pathologist.

| Case 64 | Subacute Combined Degeneration of the Spinal Cord |

Instruction

Carry out a neurological examination of this patient's legs.

Salient features

- Absent ankle jerks.
- Brisk knee jerks.
- Upgoing plantars.
- Diminished light touch, vibration and posterior column signs.
- Romberg's sign is positive.

- Examine the following:
  Mucous membranes for anaemia (pernicious anaemia).
  Abdomen for scars of previous gastrectomy (carcinoma of stomach).
  Pupils (Argyll Robertson pupil since tabes is a differential diagnosis).
  Fundus for optic atrophy, seen in this condition.
- Tell the examiner that you would like to do the following investigations:
  Take a family history of pernicious anaemia.
  Do a mini mental state examination for dementia.
  Take a history of alcohol consumption and previous gastrectomy.
  Take a history of chronic diarrhoea.

Questions

Mention a few causes of vitamin B_{12} deficiency.
- Vegan.
- Impaired absorption:
  From the stomach (pernicious anaemia, gastrectomy).
  From the small bowel (ileal disease, bacterial overgrowth, coeliac disease).
  From the pancreas (chronic pancreatic disease).
  As a result of fish tapeworm (rare).

If this patient had a haemoglobin of $6 \, g \, dl^{-1}$ how would you treat it?

I would avoid giving packed cells before replacing vitamin B_{12} as this may irreversibly exacerbate the neurological manifestations. Furthermore, blood transfusion is reported to precipitate incipient heart failure and death.

How would you investigate such a patient?

- FBC and reticulocyte count.
- Vitamin B_{12} and folate concentrations.
- Serum ferritin levels (since associated iron deficiency is common).
- Bone marrow examination.
- Parietal cell and intrinsic factor antibodies.
- Schilling test.

What type of anaemia may be seen in such patients?

Macrocytic anaemia.

Mention a few other causes of macrocytic anaemia.

- With megaloblastic bone marrow: vitamin B_{12} deficiency, folate deficiency.
- With normoblastic marrow: haemolytic anaemias, post haemorrhagic anaemias, severe hypoxia, myxoedema, hypopituitarism, bone marrow infiltration, acute leukaemia and aplastic anaemia.

What do you know about intrinsic factor antibodies?

Intrinsic factor antibodies are seen in about 50% of patients with pernicious anaemia. There are two types of antibody: type 1 – the blocking antibody – prevents vitamin B_{12} from binding to intrinsic factor, and occurs in 55% of patients; type 2 – the binding or precipitating antibody – reacts with the intrinsic factor or with the vitamin B_{12}–intrinsic factor complex, and is seen in 35% of patients. About 45% of the patients have no antibody to intrinsic factor.

What is the relationship between pernicious anaemia and gastric carcinoma?

The incidence of gastric carcinoma in patients with pernicious anaemia is increased threefold compared to the general population.

What gastrointestinal investigations would you do in an asymptomatic patient with pernicious anaemia?

In the absence of gastrointestinal symptoms a gastroscopy or a barium meal is not indicated, although many physicians tend to perform one of these investigations.

What do you understand by 'combined' degeneration of the cord?

It refers to the combined demyelination of both pyramids (or lateral columns) and posterior columns of the spinal cord.

What is the response of the neurological lesions to vitamin B_{12}?

The response to vitamin B_{12} therapy is variable: it may improve, remain unchanged or even deteriorate. Sensory abnormalities improve more than motor abnormalities and peripheral neuropathy responds to treatment better than myelopathy.

Case 65	Tabes Dorsalis

Instruction

Examine this patient's eyes.
This patient presented with lightning pains (note lightning denotes that the pains are fleeting and does not necessarily mean that they are excruciating).

Salient features

- Examine the eyes:

    Bilateral ptosis with frontalis overaction.
    Argyll Robertson pupil (irregular, small pupil which reacts sluggishly to light as compared with accommodation).
    Optic atrophy.

- Examine the sensory system:

    Posterior column signs.
    Look for loss of pain sensation but with normal touch and temperature sensation over the nose, cheeks, inner aspects of arms and legs, a band across the nipple and in the anal area.

Look for deep sensation over the Achilles tendon.

- Examine the ankle jerks (absent) and plantar response (normal).
- Examine the gait for ataxia and Romberg's sign.
- Examine knees and hips for Charcot's joints.
- Examine the feet for trophic ulcers.
- Ask the examiner if you may ask the patient about bladder sensation and impotence.

Note.

- The patient may appear older than his or her years and underweight.
- The diagnosis of neurosyphilis is based on clinical findings and examination of the serum and CSF.

Questions

What do you know about neurosyphilis?

There are five clinical patterns of neurosyphilis:

- Meningovascular disease, which occurs 3–4 years after primary infection.
- Tabes dorsalis, which occurs 10–35 years after primary infection.
- Generalised paralysis of the insane (GPI), which occurs 10–15 years after primary infection.
- Tabo paresis (a combination of the latter two).
- Localised gummata.

Tertiary syphilis of the nervous system never develops in those who have received appropriate therapy in the early stages.

What is the underlying pathology?

It is due to a combination of neuronal degeneration and/or arterial lesions.

How would you confirm the diagnosis?

The Wassermann reaction, Veneral Disease Reference Laboratory (VDRL) or Treponema pallidum haemagglutination assay (TPHA):
Meningovascular syphilis: 70% positive, whereas CSF shows 90% positive.
Tabes dorsalis: 75% positive.
GPI: nearly 100% positive.

Mention a few conditions for which the Wassermann reaction may be falsely positive.

Rheumatoid arthritis, SLE, chronic active hepatitis, infectious mononucleosis.

How would you treat the active syphilitic infection?

A course of parenteral penicillin.

In which group of patients is syphilis now common?

In those with underlying human immunodeficiency virus (HIV) infection.

What is the Jarisch–Herxheimer reaction?

An acute hypersensitivity reaction seen when a patient with syphilis is treated with penicillin. Toxins from the killed spirochaetes cause this reaction which can be fatal. Steroids are often given during the first few days of penicillin therapy.

How can this patient present to the surgeons?

With acute abdominal pain (lancinating pains).

AP von Wassermann (1866–1925), German physician.
A Jarisch (1850–1902), Professor of Dermatology in Austria.
K Herxheimer (1861–1944), Jewish German dermatologist who died in a concentration camp.

References

Hook III, EW & Marra, CM (1992) Acquired syphilis in Adults. *N Engl J Med* **326:** 1060.
Simon, RP (1985) Neurosyphilis. *Arch Neurol* **42:** 606.

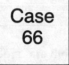

Ulnar Nerve Palsy

Instruction

Carry out a neurological examination of this patient's upper limbs.

Salient features

- Generalised wasting of the small muscles of the hand.
- There may be features of the ulnar claw hand, i.e. hyperextension at the metacarpophalangeal joints and flexion at the interphalangeal joints of the fourth and fifth fingers.
- There is weakness of movement of the fingers, except that of the thenar eminence.
- There is sensory loss over the medial one and half fingers.

- Examine the elbows for scars or signs of osteoarthroses.

Questions

What are the muscles supplied by the ulnar nerve?

In the forearm:
Flexor carpi ulnaris.
Medial half of the flexor digitorum profundus.
In the hand: Movers of the little finger – abductor digit minimi, flexor digiti minimi, opponens digiti minimi.
Adductor pollicis.
Dorsal and palmar interossei.
Third and fourth lumbricals.

Note. Remember that the ulnar nerve controls fine movements of the hand.

How would you differentiate between a lesion above the cubital fossa and a lesion at the wrist?

- In lesions above the cubital fossa the flexor carpi ulnar is involved.
- In lesions at the wrist the adductor pollicis is involved.

How would you test the flexor carpi ulnaris?

Ask the patient to keep the hand flat on a table with the palm facing upwards and then ask him to perform flexion and ulnar deviation at the wrist.

How would you test the adductor pollicis?

Ask the patient to grip a folded newspaper between thumb and index finger of each hand so that the thumbs are uppermost – this causes the adductor to contract. When the muscle is paralysed, the thumb, incapable of adequate adduction, becomes flexed at the interphalangeal joint due to contraction of the flexor pollicis longus (innervated by the median nerve). This is known as Froment's sign.

What is ulnar paradox?

The higher the lesion in the upper limb, the lesser is the deformity.

A lesion at or above the elbow causes paralysis of the ulnar half of the flexor digitorum profundus, interossei and lumbricals. Thus the action of the paralysed profundus is not unopposed by the interossei and lumbricals; as a result the little and ring fingers are not flexed and hence there is no claw.

Note. A lesion at the wrist causes an ulnar claw hand.

What causes an ulnar claw hand?

A lesion of the ulnar nerve at the wrist. The little and ring fingers are flexed at the interphalangeal joints and hyperextended at the metacarpophalangeal joints. The index and middle fingers are less affected as the first and second lumbricals are supplied by the median nerve.

What are the causes of a claw hand?

True claw hand is seen in the following conditions:
Advanced rheumatoid arthritis.
Lesion of both the median and ulnar nerves, as in leprosy.
Lesions of the medial cord of the brachial plexus.
Anterior poliomyelitis.
Syringomyelia.
Polyneuritis.
Amyotrophic lateral sclerosis.
Klumpke's paralysis.
Severe Volkmann's ischaemic contracture.

How would you rapidly exclude an injury to a major nerve in the arm?

- Radial nerve: test for wrist drop.
- Ulnar nerve: test for Froment's sign (see above).
- Median nerve: Ochsner's clasping test.

Jules Froment (1876–1946), Professor of Clinical Medicine, Lyons, France.
AJ Ochsner (b. 1896), a US surgeon, also investigated the role of tobacco in lung cancer.
Augusta Dejerine-Klumpke (1859–1927), a French neurologist, was the first woman to receive the title 'Internes des Hôpitaux' in 1877.
R von Volkmann (1830–1889), Professor of Surgery in Halle, Germany.

Case 67	Lateral Popliteal Nerve Palsy (L4, L5) (Common Peroneal Nerve Palsy)

Instruction

Examine this patient's legs.
Test this patient's gait.

Salient features

- Wasting of the muscles on the lateral aspect of the leg, namely the peronei and tibialis anterior muscle.
- Weakness of dorsiflexion and eversion of the foot.
- Foot drop.
- High steppage gait.
- Loss of sensation on the lateral aspect of the leg and dorsum of the foot.

Note. Test the ankle jerk:
　Absent ankle jerk: suspect an S1 lesion.
　Normal jerk: common peroneal nerve palsy.
　Brisk jerk: suspect an upper motor neuron lesion.

Questions

Mention a few causes.

- Compression, resulting from application of a tourniquet, or plaster of Paris casts.
- Direct trauma to the nerve.
- Leprosy.

How would you manage such patients?

- Nerve conduction studies.
- If the nerve is severed: surgery.
- If nerve is intact and concussed: 90-degree splint at night, calliper shoes with 90-degree stop, and galvanic or faradic stimulation to maintain the bulk of the muscle until the nerve recovers.

What other types of nerve injury do you know?

- Neurapraxia, i.e. concussion of the nerve after which complete recovery occurs.
- Axonotmesis, in which the axon is severed but the myelin sheath is intact; recovery may occur.
- Neurotmesis, in which the nerve is completely severed and the prognosis for recovery is poor.

What are the other causes of a foot drop?

- Peripheral neuropathy.
- L4, L5 root lesion.
- Motor neuron disease.
- Sciatic nerve palsy.
- Lumbosacral plexus lesion.

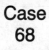

Case 68

Carpal Tunnel Syndrome

Instruction

Examine this patient's hands.

Salient features

- Wasting of the thenar eminence.
- Weakness of flexion, abduction and opposition of thumb.
- Diminished sensation over lateral three and half fingers.
- Look carefully for scar of previous surgery (hidden by the crease of the wrist).

- Percuss over the course of median nerve in the forearm: patient may experience tingling – this is Tinel's sign.

- Ask the patient to hyperextend the wrist maximally for a minute and this may bring on symptoms (dysaesthesiae over the thumb and lateral two and half fingers).
- Tell the examiner that you would like to examine for underlying causes such as myxoedema, acromegaly and rheumatoid arthritis.

Questions

How would you confirm the diagnosis?

Nerve conduction studies (increased latency at the wrist).

Mention a few causes.

- Pregnancy.
- Oral contraceptives.
- Rheumatoid arthritis.
- Myxoedema.
- Acromegaly.
- In chronic renal failure patients on long-term dialysis it is due to β_2-microglobulin as amyloid deposition.

How would you treat this condition?

- Diuretics.
- Splint.
- Local hydrocortisone.
- Surgical decompression.

■ Mention a few clinical diagnostic tests.

- Wrist extension test: the patient is asked to extend his or her wrists for a minute and this should produce numbness or tingling in the distribution of the median nerve.
- Phalen's test: the patient is asked to keep both hands with wrist in complete palmar flexion for a minute and this produces numbness or tingling in the distribution of the median nerve.
- Tourniquet test: the symptoms are produced when the blood pressure cuff is inflated above the systolic.
- Pressure test: if the pressure is placed where the median nerve leaves the carpal tunnel it causes pain.
- Luthy's sign: if the skin fold between the thumb and index finger did not close tightly around a bottle or a cup due to thumb abduction paresis, this test was regarded as positive.

Mention a few other entrapment neuropathies.

- Thoracic outlet syndromes.

- Meralgia paraesthetica (lateral cutaneous nerve of thigh trapped under the inguinal ligament).
- Elbow tunnel syndrome (ulnar nerve trapped in the cubital tunnel).
- Common peroneal nerve entrapment (pressure at the head of the fibula).
- Morton's metatarsalgia (trapped medial and lateral plantar nerves causing pain between the third and fourth toes).
- Tarsal tunnel syndrome (posterior tibial nerve is trapped).
- Suprascapular nerve trapped in the spinoglenoid notch.
- Radial nerve trapped in the humeral groove.
- Anterior interosseous nerve trapped between the heads of the pronator muscle.

Jules Tinel (1879–1952), a French neurologist, described it as the 'sign of formication' in his book on nerve wounds. He took an active part in the French Resistance.
TG Morton (1835–1903), a US surgeon, described this syndrome in 1876.

References

DeKrom, MCTF, Knipschild, PG, Kester, ADM & Spaans, F (1990) Efficacy of provocative tests for diagnosis of carpal tunnel syndrome. *Lancet* **335**: 393.

Case 69	Radial Nerve Palsy (C6–8, T1)

Instruction

Perform a neurological examination of this patient's arms.

Salient features

- There is weakness of extension of the wrist and elbow (wrist flexion is normal).

- The patient is unable to straighten his or her fingers.
- However, if the wrist is passively extended, the patient is able to straighten his or her fingers at the interphalangeal joints (due to the action of interossei and lumbricales) but is unable to extend the metacarpophalangeal joint.
- There appears to be a weakness in abduction and adduction of the fingers, but this is not present when the hand is kept flat on a table and the fingers are extended.

- Test the brachioradialis, looking for weakened elbow flexion. When the patient attempts to flex the elbow against resistance, the brachioradialis no longer springs up.
- Test triceps.
- Check sensation over first dorsal interosseous.

Remember that the radial nerve gives off two branches at the elbow:

- Superficial radial (entirely sensory).
- Posterior interosseus (entirely muscular).

- If the injury is situated above the junction of upper and middle thirds of the humerus, the action of the triceps is lost.
- If the lesion is situated in the middle third of the humerus (frequent site of fracture of the humerus), the brachioradialis is spared.

Questions

What is the cutaneous supply of the radial nerve?

Due to overlap in the areas supplied by the median and ulnar nerves only a small area of skin over the first dorsal interosseous is exclusively supplied by the radial nerve.

What are common causes of radial nerve palsy?

- An intoxicated person sleeping with his or her head resting in his or her upper arm, causing compression of the nerve over the middle third of the humerus; this is known as Saturday night palsy.
- Trauma to the nerve while it courses through the axilla, e.g. crutch palsy.

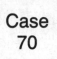

Case 70 Chorea

Instruction

Look at this patient.

Salient features

- Irregular, jerking, ill-sustained, unpredictable, quasipurposive movements of the upper limbs.
- The patient is clumsy. Mild cases may show increased fidgeting or restlessness.
- Look at the tongue for any involuntary movements – known as 'jack-in-the-box' tongue.
- Tell the examiner that you would like to make the following enquiries:
  Ask about sore throats if the patient is an adolescent, particularly if the patient is a girl; suspect Sydenham's chorea (St Vitus' dance) in rheumatic fever.
  Take a family history (especially in a middle-aged adult) of Huntington's chorea.
  Take a history of oral contraceptives in a young woman.

Questions

Mention a few more causes of chorea.

- SLE.
- Polycythaemia rubra vera.
- Chorea gravidarum, seen in pregnancy.
- Idiopathic hypoparathyroidism.
- Following a stroke.
- Kernicterus.

What is the prognosis in Sydenham's chorea?

Most patients recover within a month. A few may have relapses. A small proportion may develop valvular heart disease and hence should receive penicillin prophylaxis to prevent recurrence of rheumatic fever.

What do you know about Huntington's chorea?

It is an autosomal dominant disorder with full penetrance characterised by progressive chorea and dementia in middle life.

The defect is on the G8 locus of the chromosome 4. There is a marked reduction in acetylcholine and γ-aminobutyric acid (GABA) activity in the corpus striatum, whereas dopamine activity is normal.

George Summer Huntington (1851–1916) first documented (1909) the clinical and hereditary features of this condition in a family from Suffolk settled in Long Island in New York.

Thomas Sydenham (1624–1689) was a Puritan from Dorset and in 1666 published his first work on fevers which he dedicated to Robert Boyle.

Case 71   Hemiballismus

Instruction

Look at this patient.

Salient features

- Unilateral, involuntary, flinging movements of the proximal upper limb.

Questions

Where is the lesion?

Ipsilateral subthalamic nucleus of Luys.

What is the underlying cause?

- Vascular event, usually an infarct.
- Rarely a tumour.

What investigations would you do?

- ECG for atrial fibrillation.
- CT scan but this is usually unhelpful since the lesion is small.

What is the prognosis?

The prognosis for recovery is usually good and most patients recover within a month.

Which drug is usually used in ameliorating this condition?

Tetrabenazine.

JB Luys (1828–1897), French neurologist who also studied insanity, hysteria and hypnotism.

| Case 72 | Orofacial Dyskinesia |

Instruction

Look at this patient.

Salient features

- Smacking, chewing or chomping movement of the lips seen particularly in elderly patients; it usually involves the masticatory, lower facial and tongue muscles.
- Tell the examiner that you would like to take a drug history, in particular for phenothiazines, L-dopa and related drugs.

Questions

What is Meige's syndrome?

A combination of blepharospasm, oromandibular dystonia and cranial dystonia. There is spastic dysarthria when the throat and respiratory muscles are affected. The neck muscles are invariably involved.

What do you understand by tardive dyskinesia?

It is a drug-induced dyskinesia which appears long after drug therapy has been discontinued. It is troublesome and may resist all forms of treatment.

How would you manage such patients?

Anticholinergic drugs, baclofen, benzodiazepines and tetrabenazine but pharmacotherapy is usually ineffective.

Injection of botulinum toxin into the masseter, temporalis and internal pterygoid muscles results in an improvement in chewing and speech in approximately 80% of patients with jaw closure due to oromandibular dystonia.

Mention a few other dystonias.

Blepharospasm, spasmodic torticollis, laryngeal dystonias, writer's cramp.

H Meige (1866–1940), a French physician, also wrote on ancient Egyptian diseases.

References

Scott, AB, Kennedy, EG & Stubbs, HA (1987) Use of botulinum toxin in the treatment of 100 patients with facial dyskinesias. *Ophthalmology* 2: 237–254.

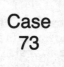

Case 73 | Internuclear Ophthalmoplegia

Instruction

Examine this patient's eyes.
Test eye movements.

Salient features

- Nystagmus is more prominent in the abducting eye (Harris's sign).
- Divergent squint.
- Abduction in either eye is normal, whereas adduction is impaired, i.e. there is dissociation of eye movements. On covering the abducting eye the adduction in the other eye is normal.

- Tell the examiner that you would like to look for other signs of demyelination – optic atrophy, pale discs, pyramidal signs.

Questions

Where is the lesion?

In the medial longitudinal bundle which connects the sixth nerve nucleus on one side to the third nerve nucleus on the opposite side of the brain stem. The eye will not adduct since the third nerve and, therefore, the medial rectus have been disconnected from the lateral gaze centre and sixth nucleus of the opposite side.

What are the causes?

- Multiple sclerosis.
- Vascular disease.
- Tumour.

How would you investigate?

- MRI scan.
- Edrophonium (Tensilon) test to exclude myasthenia.

What do you know about the 'one and a half syndrome'?

It is a syndrome in which horizontal eye movement is absent and the other eye is only capable of abduction – one and a half movements are paralysed. The vertical eye movements and the pupils are normal. The cause is a lesion in the pontine region involving the medial longitudinal fasciculus and the parapontine reticular formation on the same side. This results in failure of conjugate gaze to the same side, impairment of adduction of the eye and nystagmus on abduction of the other eye.

Case 74   Cerebellopontine Angle Tumour

Instruction

Examine this patient's cranial nerves.

Salient features

- Damage to seventh and eighth cranial nerves is the hallmark of this lesion in this region.
- Check corneal reflex and test the trigeminal nerve (see page 57).
- Tell the examiner that you would like to look for the following:
    Cerebellar signs (see page 80).
    Signs of neurofibroma type 2 (see page 123).
    Papilloedema (seen uncommonly due to raised intracranial pressure).

Questions

Mention a few causes of cerebellopontine angle lesions.

- Acoustic neuromas.

- Meningiomas, cholesteatomas, haemangioblastomas, aneurysms of the basilar artery.
- Pontine glioma.
- Medulloblastomas and astrocytomas of the cerebellum.
- Carcinoma of the nasopharynx.
- Local meningeal involvement by syphilis or tuberculosis.

What do you understand by the term 'cerebellopontine angle'?

It is the shallow triangular fossa lying between the cerebellum, lateral pons and the inner third of the petrous temporal bone. It extends from the trigeminal nerve (above) to the glossopharyngeal nerve (below). The abducens nerve runs along the medial edge, whereas the facial and auditory cranial nerves traverse the angle to enter the internal auditory meatus.

How would you investigate such patients?

- Skull X-ray, tomograms of the internal auditory meatus, and CT head scan.
- Serology for syphilis.
- Audiogram.
- Caloric test (which will reveal that the labyrinth is destroyed).
- Vertebral angiography.
- CSF may be normal or have raised protein.

Case 75   Jugular Foramen Syndrome

Instruction

Examine this patient's cranial nerves.

Salient features

- Sluggish movement of the palate when the patient says 'aah' on the affected side.

- Absent gag reflex on the same side.
- Flattening of the shoulder on the same side.
- Wasting of the sternocleidomastoid.
- Weakness when the patient moves his or her chin to the opposite side.
- Difficulty in shrugging the shoulder on the same side.

- Look for wasting and deviation of the tongue (twelfth cranial nerve palsy).
- Tell the examiner that you would like to check for two signs:
  Bovine cough.
  Husky voice.

Questions

Where is the jugular foramen located?

Between the lateral part of the occipital bone and the petrous portion of the temporal bones.

Which cranial nerves leave the skull through the jugular foramen?

The ninth, tenth and eleventh cranial nerves.

Through which foramen does the twelfth cranial nerve leave the skull?

The anterior condylar foramen.

Mention a few causes of jugular foramen syndrome.

- Carcinoma of the pharynx is the commonest cause.
- Fractured base of skull.
- Paget's disease.
- Basal meningitis.
- Neurofibroma or any tumour.
- Thrombosis of jugular vein.

Do you know of any eponymous syndromes of the lower cranial nerves?

- Vernet's syndrome: paresis of the ninth, tenth and eleventh cranial nerves due to extension of tumour into the jugular foramen.
- Collet–Sicard syndrome: fracture of the floor of the posterior cranial fossa, causing palsy of the last four cranial nerves.
- Villaret's syndrome: ipsilateral paralysis of last four cranial nerves and cervical sympathetics.

What is the cause of unilateral eleventh cranial nerve palsy?

• Trauma to the nerve in the neck.
• In hemiplegias.

How would you test for eleventh cranial nerve palsy?

• Sternocleidomastoids are tested by having the patient to turn his or head forcibly against the examiner's hand in a direction away from the muscle being tested while the muscle is observed and palpated.
• Upper portion of the trapezii are tested by having the patient forcibly elevate (shrug) his or her shoulder while the examiner attempts to depress the shoulders.

M Vernet (b. 1887), a French neurologist, described this syndrome in 1916.
M Villaret (1877–1946), a Professor of Neurology in France, described this syndrome in 1918.
FJ Collet (b. 1870), a French otolaryngologist, described his patient in 1915.
JA Sicard (1872–1929), a French physician and radiologist, was the first to do a myelogram, use alcohol in trigeminal neuralgia and inject a sclerosing substance in varicose veins. He described his patient in 1917.

References

Davis, JN, Thomas, PK, Spalding, JMK et al (1975) Diseases of the ninth, tenth and eleventh cranial nerves. In Dyck, PJ, Thomas, PK & Lambert, EH (eds) *Peripheral Neuropathy*, vol 1, pp 614–627. Philadelphia: WB Saunders.

Case 76	Pseudobulbar Palsy

Instruction

Examine this patient's cranial nerves.

Salient features

• Spastic tongue.

- Donald Duck speech.
- Patient is emotionally labile.
- Sluggish movements of the palate when the patient is asked to say 'aah'.

- Check the jaw jerk.
- Tell the examiner that you would like to do the following:
    Ask the patient whether he or she has difficulty in swallowing or nasal regurgitation.
    Check the gag reflex.
    Look for upper motor neuron signs in the limbs.

Questions

What could be the underlying cause?

- Bilateral stroke.
- Multiple sclerosis.
- Motor neuron disease.

How would you differentiate bulbar palsy from pseudobulbar palsy?

	Pseudobulbar palsy	Bulbar palsy
Prevalence	Common	Rare
Type of lesion	Upper motor neuron	Lower motor neuron, muscular
Site of lesion	Bilateral lesions, usually in the internal capsule	Medulla oblongata
Tongue	Small, stiff and spastic	Flaccid, fasciculations
Speech	Slow, thick and indistinct	Nasal twang
Nasal regurgitation	Not prominent	Prominent
Jaw jerk	Brisk	Normal or absent
Other findings	Upper motor neuron lesions of the limbs	Lower motor neuron lesions of the limbs
Affect	Emotionally labile	Normal affect
Causes	Stroke, multiple sclerosis, motor neuron disease, Creutzfeld–Jakob disease	Motor neuron disease, poliomyelitis, Guillain–Barré syndrome, myasthenia gravis, myopathy

How would you manage the swallowing and speech difficulties?

The patient would initially require assessment by a speech therapist for the difficulty in swallowing and speech deficits. Barium swallow with videofluoroscopy may be required in order to 'visualise' the swallowing.

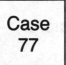

Case 77 | Bulbar Palsy

Instruction

Examine this patient's cranial nerves.
Ask him or her a few questions.
Test this patient's speech.

Salient features

- Nasal speech lacking in modulation and patient has great difficulty with all consonants.
- Wasting of the tongue with fasciculations.
- Weakness of soft palate: ask the patient to say 'aah'.
- There may be accumulation of saliva.

- Check the jaw jerk (normal or absent).
- Tell the examiner that you would like to do the following:
    Ask the patient about nasal regurgitation, dysphagia.
    Check the gag reflex.
    Examine the hands for fasciculations, dissociated sensory loss.

Questions

What may be the underlying cause?

- Motor neuron disease (see page 121).
- Guillain–Barré syndrome.
- Syringomyelia (see page 125).
- Poliomyelitis.
- Nasopharyngeal tumours.
- Neurosyphilis.
- Neurosarcoid.

C Guillain (1876–1961), Professor of Medicine, Paris.
JA Barré (1800–1967), Professor of Neurology in Strasbourg, trained in Paris.

Case 78	Wallenberg's Syndrome (Lateral Medullary Syndrome)

Instruction

Examine this patient's cranial nerves.

Salient features

- Nystagmus.
- Ipsilateral involvement of fifth, sixth, seventh and eighth cranial nerves.
- Bulbar palsy: impaired gag, sluggish palatal movements.
- Horner's syndrome.

- Tell the examiner that you would like to check for the following:
    Cerebellar signs on the same side.
    Pain and temperature sensory loss on the opposite side.

Questions

Which vessel is occluded?

Any of the following five vessels:
    Posterior inferior cerebellar artery.
    Vertebral artery.
    Superior, middle or inferior lateral medullary arteries.

How may these patients present?

With sudden onset of vertigo, vomiting and ipsilateral ataxia with contralateral loss of pain and temperature sensation.

What is the medial medullary syndrome?

It is caused by occlusion of the lower basilar artery or vertebral artery. Ipsilateral lesions result in paralysis and wasting of the tongue. Contralateral lesions result in hemiplegia and loss of vibration and joint position sense.

Mention a few other eponymous syndromes with crossed hemiplegias.

- Weber's syndrome: contralateral hemiplegia with ipsilateral lower motor neuron lesion of the oculomotor nerve. The lesion is in the midbrain.
- Millard–Gubler syndrome: contralateral hemiplegia with lower motor neuron of the abducens nerve. The lesion is in the pons.
- Foville's syndrome: as Millard–Gubler with gaze palsy.

What is Benedikt's syndrome?

It causes cerebellar signs opposite the third nerve palsy (which is produced by damage to the nucleus itself or to the nerve fascicle). It is due to a midbrain vascular lesion causing damage to the red nucleus, interrupting the dentatorubrothalamic tract from the opposite cerebellar signs.

Auguste LJ Millard (1830–1915) and Adolphe Marie Gubler (1821–1879), Paris physicians.
Achille LF Foville (1799–1878), Paris neurologist.
A Wallenberg (1862–1949), a German neurologist, described his syndrome in 1895.

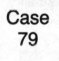 **Case 79**   **Winging of Scapula**

Instruction

Look at this patient's back.

Salient features

- Winging of the scapula.
- Difficulty in raising the arm above the horizontal.

- Check whether it is unilateral or bilateral.

- Ask the patient to push the outstretched arm firmly against your hand and check whether or not the winging is more prominent.
- Tell the examiner that you would like to examine the muscles in the arm to rule out muscular dystrophy.

Questions

Which nerve lesion is responsible for these signs?

Long thoracic nerve of Bell arising from the anterior rami of C5, C6, and C7.

Which muscle is supplied by this nerve?

Serratus anterior.

What is the action of the serratus anterior?

It is responsible for the lateral and forward movement of the scapula, keeping it closely applied to the thorax.

Which other muscle palsy can cause winging of the scapula?

Paralysis of the trapezius.

How would you differentiate winging of the scapula caused by serratus anterior palsy from that of trapezius palsy?

In serratus anterior palsy abduction of the arm laterally produces little winging of the scapula, whereas winging due to weakness of the trapezius is intensified by abduction of the arm against resistance.

RESPIRATORY SYSTEM

Examination of the Chest

1. Introduce yourself to the patient.

2. Place the patient in a sitting position and ask if he or she is comfortable.

3. Examine the sputum cup.

4. Examine the patient from the foot end of the bed and comment as follows:
   - Whether the patient is breathless at rest.
   - On wasting, if any, in the infraclavicular region.
   - On diminished movement on right or left side.
   - Count respiratory rate.

5. Examine the hands:
   - Clubbing.
   - Cyanosis.
   - Tar staining (the yellow 'nicotine' staining is actually due to tar).
   - Examine the pulse for bounding pulse and asterixis (signs of carbon monoxide narcosis).

6. Examine the face:
   - Comment on the tongue, looking for central cyanosis.
   - Comment on the eyes, looking for pallor and evidence of Horner's syndrome.

7. Examine the neck:
   - Comment on the neck veins.
   - Check for cervical lymphadenopathy.
   - Comment on the trachea:
     Whether or not it is deviated.
     The distance between the cricoid cartilage and suprasternal notch.

8. Palpate:
   - Apex beat.
   - Movements on both sides with the fingers symmetrically placed in the intercostal spaces on both sides.
   - Vocal fremitus (tell the examiner that you would prefer to do vocal resonance since it gives the same information and is more reliable).

9. Percussion:
   - Percuss over supraclavicular areas, clavicles, upper, middle and lower chest on both sides.

10. Auscultate:
    - Over supraclavicular areas, upper, middle and lower chest on both sides – comment on breath sounds (whether vesicular or bronchial) and on adventitious sounds (wheeze, crackles or pleural rub). If crackles are heard ask the patient to cough and then repeat auscultation. It is important to time the crackles to ascertain whether they are early, mid or late inspiration.
    - Check for vocal resonance by asking the patient to repeat 'one, one, one'.
    - Check for forced expiratory time (FET) if your diagnosis is chronic obstructive airways disease (COAD) by asking the patient to exhale forcefully after full inspiration while you are listening over the trachea: if patient takes more than 6 seconds, airways disease is indicated.

11. Ask the patient to sit forward:
    - Palpate – assess expansion posteriorly.
    - Percuss – on both sides including the axillae.
    - Auscultate – posteriorly including the axillae.

12. Remember to look for signs of middle lobe disease in the right axilla.

Case 80	Pleural Effusion

Instruction

Examine this patient's chest.
Examine this patient's chest from the back.
Examine this patient's chest from the front.

Salient features

- Decreased movement on the affected side.
- Tracheal deviation to the opposite side.
- Stony dull note on the affected side.
- Decreased vocal resonance and diminished breath sounds on the affected side.

- It is important to elicit any evidence of an underlying cause, such as clubbing, tar staining, lymph nodes, radiation burns and mastectomy, raised JVP, rheumatoid hands, butterfly rash.
- Comment on aspiration marks:
  Percuss for the upper level of the effusion in the axilla.
  Listen for bronchial breath sounds.
- Listen for aegophony at the upper level of the effusion.

Questions

How would you investigate this patient?

CXR and pleural tap for proteins and cytology; pleural biopsy.

What are the causes of dullness at a lung base?

- Pleural effusion.
- Pleural thickening.
- Consolidation and collapse of the lung.
- Raised hemidiaphragm.

How would you differentiate between the above?

- Pleural effusion: stony dull note; trachea may be deviated to the opposite side in large effusions.

- Pleural thickening: trachea not deviated; breath sounds will be heard.
- Consolidation: vocal resonance increased; bronchial breath sounds and associated crackles.
- Collapse: trachea deviated to the affected side; absent breath sounds.

How would you differentiate between an exudate and a transudate?

The protein content of an exudate is more than $3\,g\,l^{-1}$. However, if this criterion alone is applied, about 10% of the exudates and 15% of the transudates will be wrongly classified. A more accurate diagnosis is made when the following criteria for an exudate are applied: (1) the ratio of pleural fluid to serum protein is greater than 0.5 and (2) the ratio of pleural fluid to serum lactic dehydrogenase (LDH) is greater than 0.6.

Mention a few causes for an exudate and a transudate.

- Causes of an exudate:
    Bronchogenic carcinoma.
    Secondaries in the pleura.
    Pneumonia.
    Pulmonary infarction.
    Tuberculosis.
    Rheumatoid arthritis.
    SLE.
    Lymphoma.
    Mesothelioma.
- Causes of a transudate:
    Nephrotic syndrome.
    Cardiac failure.
    Liver cell failure.
    Hypothyroidism.

What further investigation would you do to determine the underlying cause of the pleural effusion?

Pleural biopsy.

■ What characteristics of the pleural fluid in a parapneumonic effusion indicate a need for closed-tube drainage?

A pleural fluid glucose less than $40\,mg\,dl^{-1}$ or a pH <7.0 indicates a need for closed-tube drainage.

What does a pleural fluid total neutral fat greater than 400 mg dl^{-1} suggest?

It suggests a chylothorax and is seen most often with lymphomas, solid tumours, nephrotic syndrome and cirrhosis, and occasionally in rheumatoid arthritis.

What is the significance of pleural fluid amylase levels?

Pleural fluid amylase when greater than amylase is seen in pancreatitis, lung carcinoma, bacterial pneumonias and oesophageal rupture.

In which conditions is the pleural fluid bloody?

Haemorrhagic fluid is seen in malignancy, pulmonary embolus, tuberculosis and trauma to the chest.

What are the earliest X-ray signs of pleural fluid?

The earliest radiological signs are blunting of the costophrenic angle on the anterior–posterior view or loss of clear definition of the diaphragm posteriorly on the lateral view.

When in doubt of a small effusion, how would you confirm your suspicions?

Either a lateral decubitus view (which shows a layering of the fluid along the dependent chest wall unless the fluid is loculated) or by ultrasonography.

What is a pseudotumour?

It is the accumulation of fluid between the major or minor fissure or along the lateral chest wall and can be mistaken for a tumour on the CXR. Such loculated effusions can be confirmed by using ultrasonography.

What are the complications of thoracocentesis?

Pneumothorax, haemothorax, intravascular collapse and unilateral pulmonary oedema (the latter after withdrawal of large quantities of fluid).

What do you know about Meigs' syndrome?

Meigs' syndrome comprises pleural effusion (usually right-sided and a transudate) and an ovarian malignancy (usually benign ovarian fibroma).

Mention some causes of drug-induced pleural effusion.

Practolol, procarbazine, methysergide, bromocriptine, methotrexate, nitrofurantoin.

What do you know about yellow nail syndrome?

Yellow nail syndrome is the association of primary lymphoedema with a yellow discolouration of the nails and sometimes with pleural effusion.

This patient used to be a shipbuilder – what diagnosis would you consider?

It is most likely that this patient has malignant mesothelioma and if the diagnosis is confirmed I would advise him to apply for industrial injuries benefit.

References

Hirsch, A, Ruffie, P, Nebut, M et al (1979) Pleural effusion: laboratory tests in 300 cases. *Thorax* **304:** 106.
Prakash, UBS & Reiman, HM (1985) Comparison of needle biopsy with cytologic analysis for the evaluation of pleural effusion. Analysis of 414 cases. *Mayo Clin Proc* **60:** 158.
Seaton, A (1990) Asbestos diseases and compensation. *Br Med J* **301:** 453.

Case 81	Pleural Rub

Instruction

Listen to this patient's chest.
Examine this patient's chest.
This patient presented with sudden onset of lateral chest pain aggravated by deep inspiration and coughing.

Salient features

- Pleural rub (superficial, scratchy, grating sound heard on deep inspiration).

- Differentiate between pleural rub and crackles by asking the patient to cough and check whether or not there is any change in nature. (**Note.** No change with the pleural rub.)
- Tell the examiner that you would like to proceed as follows:
   Listen for tachycardia and right ventricular gallop.
   Take a history of the nature of the sputum (purulent expectoration in a chest infection, haemoptysis in pulmonary embolism).
   Take a drug history (oral contraceptives).

Questions

What is your diagnosis?

Pleurisy, due to either underlying infection or pulmonary embolism.

How would you investigate this patient?

- FBC.
- Sputum cultures.
- Blood gases.
- ECG.
- CXR.
- Ventilation–perfusion scan.

■ What would you expect to see in the ventilation–perfusion scan in a patient with pulmonary embolism?

In acute pulmonary embolism the area of decreased perfusion usually has normal ventilation, whereas in pneumonia there are abnormalities in both the ventilation and the perfusion scan.

How would you treat a patient with pulmonary embolism?

- Initially with heparin and then with oral anticoagulants for at least 3 months.
- Pain relief for pleurisy.

| Case 82 | Asthma |

Instruction

Examine this patient's chest.

Salient features

- Bilateral scattered wheeze.
- Tell the examiner that you would like to know whether or not the following apply:
  It is reversible airway obstruction (by taking a history).
  There is a history of atopy (eczema, hay fever).

Questions

Mention a few trigger factors known to aggravate asthma.

- Infection.
- Emotion.
- Exercise.
- Drugs, e.g. beta blockers.
- External allergens.

What you understand by the term 'asthma'?

Asthma is an inflammatory disorder characterised by hyperresponsiveness of the airways to various stimuli, resulting in widespread narrowing of the airways. The changes are reversible either spontaneously or as a result of therapy.

What do you understand by the term 'intrinsic asthma'?

Intrinsic asthma is of nonallergic aetiology and usually begins after the age of 30. It tends to be more continuous and more severe; status asthmaticus is common in this group.

What do you understand by the term 'extrinsic asthma'?

Extrinsic asthma has a clearly defined history of allergy to a variety of inhaled factors and is characterised by a childhood onset and seasonal variation.

What are the indications for steriods in chronic asthma?

- Sleep is disturbed by wheeze.
- Morning tightness persists until midday.
- Symptoms and peak expiratory flows progressively deteriorate each day.
- Maximum treatment with bronchodilators.
- Emergency nebulisers are needed.

How would you manage a patient with acute asthma?

- Nebulised beta agonists e.g. terbutaline or salbutamol.
- Oxygen, using highest concentration of oxygen.
- High-dose steroids: intravenous hydrocortisone 200 mg.
- Blood gases.
- CXR to rule out pneumothorax.

What are the imminently life-threatening indicators in acute asthma?
- Cyanosis.
- Exhaustion, confusion, unconsciousness.
- Silent chest.
- Bradycardia.

What are the potentially life-threatening features of a severe attack?

- Increasing wheeze and shortness of breath so that the patient is unable to complete sentences.
- Respiratory rate greater than 25 per minute.
- Heart rate greater than 110 beats per minute.
- Peak flow less than 40% of predicted or less than 200 l per minute.
- An inspiratory fall in systolic blood pressure greater than 10 mmHg.
- Severe hypoxia less than 8 kPa.
- Normal or increased carbon dioxide tension.

In which other conditions is wheeze a prominent sign?

COAD, left ventricular failure (cardiac asthma), polyarteritis nodosa, eosinophilic lung disease, recurrent thromboembolism, tumour causing localised wheeze.

■ What are the indications for mechanical ventilation with intermittent positive pressure ventilation?

- Worsening hypoxia (Pao_2 less than 8 kPa) despite 60% inspired oxygen.

- Hypercapnia ($Paco_2$ more than 6 kPa).
- Drowsiness.
- Unconsciousness.
- Intermittent positive pressure ventilation.

Professor PJ Barnes, contemporary chest physician, National Institute for Heart and Lung Diseases, London; his major interest is asthma.

References

Ayres, JG (1990) Late onset asthma. *Br Med J* **300:** 1602.
Benetar, SR (1986) Fatal asthma. *N Engl J Med* **314:** 423.
British Thoracic Society and others (1990) Guidelines for management of asthma in adults: I & II. *Br Med J* **301:** 651, 797.
Fitzgerald, JM & Hargreave, FE (1989) The assessment and management of life threatening asthma. *Chest* **95:** 888.
Rees, PJ (1990) Guidelines for the management of asthma in adults. *Br Med J* **301:** 771.

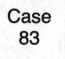

Case 83   Chronic Bronchitis or Emphysema

Instruction

Examine this patient's chest.

Salient features

- Begin with examination of the *sputum pot*.
- Observe the patient from the end of the bed – for obvious breathlessness, pursed lip breathing and symmetrical chest movements – and count respiratory rate.
- Look for nail changes such as tar staining.

- Feel the palms for warmth and feel the pulse for rapid bounding pulse (signs of carbon dioxide retention).
- Look at the lips and tongue for central cyanosis.

In the neck:

- Comment on the active contractions of the accessory muscles of respiration such as the sternocleidomastoids, scaleni and trapezii.
- Palpate for tracheal deviation and measure the distance between the cricoid cartilage and suprasternal notch (less than three fingers' breadth in emphysema).
- Comment on the raised JVP.

Palpate for:

- Apex beat.
- Chest expansion.
- Vocal fremitus.

Percussion:

- Look for hyperresonance and obliteration of cardiac and liver dullness.

Auscultate for:

- Breath sounds.
- Vocal resonance.
- FET: normal individuals can empty their chests from full inspiration in 4 seconds or less. The end point of FET is detected by auscultating over the trachea in the suprasternal notch. Prolongation of the FET to more than 6 seconds indicates airflow obstruction.

Questions

What do you understand by the term 'chronic bronchitis'?

Chronic bronchitis is cough with mucoid expectoration for at least 3 months in a year for 2 successive years.

What is the definition of emphysema?

Emphysema is the abnormal permanent enlargement of the airways distal to terminal respiratory bronchioles with destruction of their walls. Clinical, radiological and lung function tests give an imprecise picture in an individual case but a combination of all these features give a reasonable picture.

How would you differentiate emphysema from chronic bronchitis?

	Emphysema	Chronic bronchitis
	Pink puffer	Blue bloater
Cyanosis	Absent	Prominent
Dyspnoea	+ +	+
Hyperinflation	+ +	+
Cor pulmonale	—	Common
Respiratory drive	High	Low

If this patient was between the ages of 30 and 45 what would you consider to be the underlying cause for his emphysema?

Smoking, alpha-1 antitrypsin (AAT) deficiency.

How would you treat an acute exacerbation?

- Nebulised bronchodilators (terbutaline, ipratropium bromide).
- Intravenous antibiotics.
- Oxygen (24%).
- Intravenous hydrocortisone and oral steriods.

■ What clinical features would suggest that this patient is suitable for long-term domiciliary oxygen therapy?

- COAD: (forced expiratory volume in 1 second (FEV_1) less than 1.5 l; forced vital capacity (FVC) less than 2 l) and stable chronic respiratory failure (Pao_2 less than 7.3 kPa) in patients who have (1) had peripheral oedema or (2) not necessarily had hypercapnia or oedema.
- Terminally ill patients of whatever cause with severe hypoxia (Pao_2 less than 7.3 kPa).

How can the sensation of breathlessness be reduced?

By the use of either promethazine 125 mg daily or dihydrocodeine 1 mg kg^{-1} orally.

How would you treat the acute respiratory failure?

If Pao_2 is less than 8 kPa, administer 24% oxygen. There is no need for oxygen if Pao_2 is greater than 8. Monitor blood gases after 30 minutes. If Pco_2 is rising (by 1 kPa), monitor blood gases hourly. If Pco_2 continues to rise, administer doxopram. If, in spite of this, the patient continues to deteriorate, artificial ventilation may be called for.

What do you know about α_1-antitrypsin deficiency?

The patient is deficient in α_1-antitrypsin and his or her activity is approximately 15% of the normal. Concentrations of 40% or more are required for health. The patient is homozygous for protease inhibitor (Pi) ZZ gene. Other genetic combinations and their percentage of normal activities are PiMS (80%), PiMZ (60%), PiSS (60%), PiSZ (40%). Six per cent of the population is heterozygous for S(PiMS), and 4% for Z(PiMZ), making an overall frequency of 1 in 10 for the carriage of the deficient gene. Liver transplantation results in conversion to the genotype of the donor.

The emphysema is panacinar and is seen in the lower lobes of the lungs.

The siblings of an index case should be screened for this disorder. Their identification should be followed by counselling to avoid smoking and occupations with atmospheric pollution. Children of homozygotes will inherit at least one Z gene and hence will be heterozygotes. They should avoid pairing with another heterozygote to avoid the risk of producing an affected homozygote.

Mention other diseases that are treated with liver transplantation.

- Primary biliary cirrhosis.
- Wilson's disease.
- Biliary atresia.
- Primary liver tumours.
- Budd–Chiari syndrome.

Peter Howard, contemporary chest physician, Sheffield; his chief interest is long-term domiciliary oxygen therapy.

References

Flenley, DC (1986) The pathogenesis of pulmonary emphysema. *Q J Med* **61**: 901.
Howard, P & Stewart, AG (1991) Cor pulmonale and long-term domiciliary oxygen therapy. *Med Int* **89**: 3727.

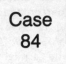

Case 84   Bronchiectasis

Instruction

Examine this patient's chest.

Salient features

- Copious purulent expectoration (remember to check the sputum cup in a chest case).
- Finger clubbing.
- Bilateral, coarse, late inspiratory crackles.

In addition there may be signs of collapse, fibrosis or pneumonia.

Questions

What do you understand by the term 'bronchiectasis'?

It is defined as the abnormal, permanent dilatation of the airways.

Mention the causes of bronchiectasis.

- Postpneumonic, measles, pertussis, TB, and others.
- Mechanical bronchial obstruction, as in TB, carcinoma, nodal compression.
- Immunological disease, allergic bronchopulmonary aspergillosis.
- γ-Globulin deficiency – congenital, acquired.
- Immotile cilia syndrome.
- Cystic fibrosis.
- Neuropathic disorders, namely Riley–Day syndrome, Chagas' disease.
- Idiopathic.

What investigations would you do in such a patient?

FBC, sputum culture, CXR, bronchography, CT scan of the chest.

What are the complications of bronchiectasis?

- Pneumonia, pleurisy, pleural effusion, pneumothorax.
- Sinusitis.

- Haemoptysis.
- Brain abscess.
- Amyloidosis.

Which are the major respiratory pathogens in bronchiectasis?

Staphylococcus aureus, Haemophilus influenzae, Pseudomonas aeruginosa.

How would you treat such patients?

- Postural drainage.
- Antibiotics.
- Bronchodilators.
- Surgery in selected cases.

What abnormalities may be associated with bronchiectasis?

- Congenital absence of bronchial cartilage (Williams–Campbell syndrome).
- Congenital kyphoscoliosis.
- Congenital heart disease (Kartagener's syndrome).
- Unilateral absence of pulmonary artery.

What is the indication for surgery in bronchiectasis?

Bronchiectasis localised to a single lobe or a segment without clinical, bronchographic or CT evidence of bronchiectasis or bronchitis affecting other parts of the lung.

Which are the common sites for localised disease?

Left lower lobe and lingula.

M Kartagener (b. 1897), Swiss physician.
CM Riley and RL Day, both American paediatricians. Riley–Day syndrome consists of dysautonomia and lack of co-ordination in swallowing.
CJR Chagas (1879–1934), Brazilian physician.

```
┌─────────┐
│  Case   │   Cor Pulmonale
│   85    │
└─────────┘
```

Instruction

Examine this patient's chest.

Salient features

- Patient is short of breath at rest and centrally cyanosed.
- Tar staining of the fingers.
- JVP is raised: both 'a' and 'v' waves are seen, 'v' waves being prominent if there is associated tricuspid regurgitation.
- There may be a right ventricular gallop rhythm.
- On examination of the chest there is bilateral wheeze and other signs of chronic bronchitis (see page 162).
- There may be left parasternal heave (often absent when the chest is barrel shaped).
- Loud P_2 and loud ejection click.
- There may be a pansystolic murmur of tricuspid regurgitation.
- There may be an early diastolic Graham Steell murmur in the pulmonary area.

- Look for signs of:
    Hepatomegaly.
    Pedal oedema.

Questions

What do you understand by the term 'cor pulmonale'?

Cor pulmonale is right ventricular enlargement due to the increase in its afterload which occurs in diseases of the lung, chest wall or pulmonary circulation.

Mention a few causes of cor pulmonale.

Respiratory disorders:

- Obstructive:
    COAD, chronic persistent asthma.

- Restrictive:
    Intrinsic – interstitial fibrosis, lung resection.
    Extrinsic – obesity, muscle weakness, kyphoscoliosis, high altitude.

Pulmonary vascular disorders:

- Pulmonary emboli.
- Vasculitis of small pulmonary arteries.
- Adult respiratory distress syndrome (ARDS).
- Primary pulmonary hypertension.

How would you manage a patient with cor pulmonale?

- Treat the underlying cause.
- Treat respiratory failure. If Pao_2 is less than 8 kPa, administer 24% oxygen. There is no need for oxygen if Pao_2 is more than 8. Monitor blood gases after 30 minutes. If Pco_2 is rising (by 1 kPa), monitor blood gases hourly. If Pco_2 continues to rise, administer doxopram. If, in spite of this, the patient continues to deteriorate, the patient may merit artificial ventilation.
- Treat cardiac failure with frusemide.
- Consider venesection if the haematocrit is more than 55%.

What is the prognosis in cor pulmonale?

Approximately 50% of patients succumb within 5 years.

References

Editorial (1989) Polycythemia due to hypoxemia: advantage or disadvantage. *Lancet* 2: 20–21.

Case 86   Consolidation

Instruction

Examine this patient's chest.

Salient features

- Purulent sputum (if bacterial in aetiology).
- Tachypnoea.
- Reduced movement of the affected side.
- Trachea central.
- Impaired percussion note.
- Bronchial breath sounds.
- Crackles.

Questions

What is the aetiology?

- Bacterial pneumonia.
- Bronchogenic carcinoma.
- Pulmonary infarct.

How would you investigate a suspected bacterial pneumonia?

- FBC.
- Sputum culture.
- Blood culture.
- Titres of legionella, mycoplasma.
- CXR.

What are the causes of a poorly resolving or recurrent pneumonia?

- Carcinoma of the lung.
- Aspiration of a foreign body.
- Inappropriate antibiotic.
- Sequestration (rare; suspect if left lower lobe is involved).

What do you know about atypical pneumonias?

Typical pneumonia is due to pneumococcus, whereas atypical pneumonia is that *not* due to pneumococcus; the latter may be due to mycoplasma, legionella, chlamydiae, coxiella, etc. The clinical picture in atypical pneumonia is dominated by constitutional symptoms, such as fever and headache, rather than by respiratory symptoms.

What do you know about mycoplasma pneumonia?

Mycoplasma pneumoniae is an important cause for atypical pneumonia. It is an important cause for community-acquired pneumonia and epidemics are seen every 4 years or so. Its incubation period is 2–3 weeks and is usually seen in children and young adults. Reinfection can occur in older patients with detectable *M. pneumoniae* antibody. Like all other pneumonias, mycoplasma pneumonia is common in winter months.

What are the extrapulmonary manifestations of mycoplasma pneumonia?

- Arthralgia and arthritis.
- Autoimmune haemolytic anaemia.
- Neurological manifestations involving both the central and peripheral systems.
- Pericarditis, myocarditis.
- Hepatitis, glomerulonephritis.
- Nonspecific rash, erythema multiforme and Stevens–Johnson syndrome.
- Disseminated intravascular coagulation (DIC).

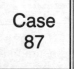

| Case 87 | Bronchogenic Carcinoma |

Instruction

Examine this patient's chest.

Salient features

- *Patient 1* has clubbing and tar staining of his or her fingers.
- Dull percussion note at the apex with absent breath sounds.
- Look for Horner's syndrome and wasting of small muscles of the hand.

- *Patient 2* has signs of pleural effusion on one side.

- *Patient 3* shows signs of unilateral collapse or consolidation of the upper lobe on one side.

- If you suspect bronchogenic carcinoma, always look for clubbing, tar staining, cervical lymph nodes and radiation marks, and comment on cachexia.

Questions

How may patients with bronchogenic carcinoma present?

- Cough (in 80% of cases), haemoptysis (70%) and dyspnoea (60%); loss of weight, anorexia.
- Skeletal manifestations: clubbing (in 30% of cases).
- Local pressure effects: recurrent laryngeal palsy, superior vena caval obstruction, Horner's syndrome.
- Endocrine manifestations (12% of tumours) – in particular, small-cell tumours – present with syndrome of inappropriate anti-diuretic hormone (SIADH), hypercalcaemia, adrenocortico-trophic hormone (ACTH) secretion, gynaecomastia.
- Neurological manifestations: Eaton–Lambert syndrome, cerebellar degeneration, polyneuropathy, dementia, proximal myopathy.
- Cardiovascular: thrombophlebitis migrans, atrial fibrillation, peri-carditis, nonbacterial thrombotic endocarditis.
- Cutaneous manifestations: dermatomyositis, acanthosis nigricans, herpes zoster.
- Anaemia, DIC, thrombotic thrombocytopenic purpura.

How would you investigate this patient?

- Sputum cytology.
- CXR.
- Pleural fluid cytology.
- Bronchoscopy.
- CT scan of the chest.
- Bone scan for metastases (helpful in staging).

■ What is the role of surgery in lung carcinoma?

Surgery is beneficial in peripheral non-small-cell carcinoma. Its role is limited in small-cell carcinoma as over 90% would have metastasised by the time of diagnosis.

Which tumours respond well to chemotherapy?

Small-cell carcinoma: cyclophosphamide, doxorubicin, etopside and vincristine are some of the drugs used.

What are the indications for radiotherapy?

- Pain – either local or metastatic.
- Breathlessness due to bronchial obstruction.
- Dysphagia.
- Haemoptysis.
- Superior vena caval obstruction.
- Pancoast's tumour.
- Preoperatively and postoperatively in selected patients.

What are the contraindications for surgery?

- Metastatic carcinoma.
- FEV_1 less than 1.5 l.
- Transfer factor less than 50%.
- Severe pulmonary hypertension.
- Uncontrolled major arrhythmias.
- Carbon dioxide retention.
- Myocardial infarction in the past 3 months.

Is the progression of cancer associated with genetic change?

Yes: it is accompanied by a mutation in the p53 gene and loss of a portion of the short arm of chromosome 3 in small-cell cancer; the functional significance of this is not clear.

Robert Souhami, Professor of Clinical Oncology, University College and Middlesex School of Medicine, London.

References

Souhami, R (1992) Lung cancer. *Br Med J* **304:** 1298.
Spiro, SG (1990) Management of lung cancer. *Br Med J* **301:** 1287.

Case 88 Cystic Fibrosis

Instruction

Examine the chest of this patient who has a good appetite, poor weight gain and foul fatty stool.

Salient features

- Sputum is purulent.
- Patient is short of breath.
- Central cyanosis.
- Finger clubbing.
- Bilateral, coarse crackles.

- Tell the examiner that you would like to check the following levels:
  Urine sugar.
  Faecal fat.
  Sweat sodium.

Questions

What are the chances of this male patient having a child?

Males are sterile owing to the failure of the development of the vas deferens and epididymis.

What are the clinical manifestations of this condition?

- Neonates recurrent chest infections, failure to thrive, meconium ileus and rectal prolapse.
- In childhood and young adults: bronchiectasis, malabsorption, meconium ileus equivalent, cirrhosis and infertility, nasal polyps.

How would you treat steatorrhoea?

- Low-fat diet.
- Pancreatic supplements.
- H_2 receptor antagonist.

How would you treat chest complications?

- Postural drainage.
- Antibiotics.
- Bronchodilators.
- Heart–lung transplantation.

■ **What is the inheritance in cystic fibrosis?**

Autosomal recessive and a specific gene deletion has been identified in 70% of patients. There is a mutation on the long arm of chromosome 7. There is a deletion of the codon for phenylalanine at position 508(Δ508). This results in a defect in a transmembrane regulator protein. This gene is carried by 1 in 20 Caucasians and its incidence is about 1 in 2000 live births.

How is this condition diagnosed in infancy?

Immunoreactive reactive trypsin assay in dried blood.

What do you know about sweat testing?

A sweat sodium concentration over 60 mmol l^{-1} is indicative of cystic fibrosis. It identifies over 75% by the age of 2 and about 95% by the age of 12. It is more difficult to interpret in older children and adults.

If the patient has persistent purulent cough which organisms are usually responsible?

Staphylococcus aureus, Haemophilus influenzae and *Pseudomonas aeruginosa.* The latter is associated with poor prognosis as this organism is almost impossible to eradicate.

Which antibiotics are usually used to treat pseudomonas infections?

Intravenous or aerosol carbenicillin and gentamicin in combination.

What is the life span in such patients?

Survival beyond the age of 30 is unusual.

What is the cause of death in cystic fibrosis?

Death occurs from pulmonary complications, such as pneumonia, pneumothorax or haemoptysis, or as a result of terminal chronic respiratory failure.

References

Davis, PB (1985) Cystic fibrosis. *Semin Respir Med* **6:** 243.
Editorial (1990) Cystic fibrosis: towards ultimate therapy, slowly. *Lancet* **336:** 1225.
Fick Jr, RB & Stillwell, PC (1989) Controversies in the management of pulmonary disease due to cystic fibrosis. *Chest* **95:** 1319.
Kerem, E, Corey, M, Kerem, B et al (1990) The relation between genotype and phenotype in cystic fibrosis – analysis of the most common mutation (ΔF 508). *N Engl J Med* **323:** 1517.

Case 89	Fibrosing Alveolitis

Instruction

Examine this patient's chest.
Examine the respiratory system from the back.

Salient features

- Clubbing (in 60% of cases).
- Central cyanosis.
- Bilateral, basal, fine, end inspiratory crackles which disappear or become quieter on leaning forwards. Furthermore, the crackles do not disappear on coughing (unlike those of pulmonary oedema). The crackles have been called 'Velcro' or 'Cellophane' crackles.
- Tachypnoea (in advanced cases).

- Examine the following:
  Hands (for rheumatoid arthritis, systemic sclerosis).
  Face (for typical rash of SLE, heliotropic rash of dermatomyositis, typical facies of systemic sclerosis, lupus pernio of sarcoid).
  Mouth (for aphthous ulcers of Crohn's disease, dry mouth of Sjögrens syndrome).
- Look for signs of pulmonary hypertension: 'a' wave in the JVP, left parasternal heave and loud P_2.

- Tell the examiner that you would like to take a drug history (amiodarone, nitrofurantoin, busulfan).

Questions

In which other conditions is clubbing associated with crackles?

- Bronchogenic carcinoma (crackles are localised).
- Bronchiectasis (coarse crackles).
- Asbestosis (history of exposure to asbestos).

Mention other conditions which have similar pulmonary changes.

- Rheumatoid arthritis, SLE, dermatomyositis, chronic active hepatitis, ulcerative colitis, systemic sclerosis.
- Pneumoconiosis.
- Granulomatous disease: sarcoid, TB.
- Chronic pulmonary oedema.
- Radiotherapy.
- Lymphangitis carcinomatosa.
- Extrinsic allergic alveolitis: farmer's lung, bird fancier's lung.

■ How would you investigate this patient?

- CXR typically shows bilateral basal reticulonodular shadows which progress upwards as the disease progresses. In advanced cases there is marked destruction of the parenchyma, causing 'honeycombing' (due to groups of closely set ring shadows), and nodular shadows are not conspicuous. The mediastinum may appear broad as a result of a decrease in lung volumes.
- Blood gases: arterial desaturation worsens while upright and improves on recumbency. There is arterial hypo-oxaemia and *hypocapnia*.
- Pulmonary function tests: in early stages lung volumes may be normal, but there is arterial desaturation following exercise. Typically there is a restrictive defect with reduction of both the gas transfer factor and the gas transfer coefficient.
- High ESR; raised immunoglobulins; raised antinuclear factor; rheumatoid factor is positive.
- Bronchial lavage: large number of lymphocytes indicates a good response to steroids and a good prognosis. A large number of neutrophils and eosinophils indicates a poor response to steroids and a poor prognosis (60% 5-year survival to steroid responders versus 25% 5-year survival to nonresponders).
- Lung biopsy: in the early stages there is mononuclear cell infiltrate in the alveolar walls, progressing to interstitial fibrosis – known as

usual interstitial pneumonitis (UIP); in the later stages, fibrotic contraction of the lung, honeycombing, bronchial dilatation and cysts are seen. Desquamative interstitial pneumonitis (DIP) – alveolar macrophages with little mononuclear infiltration or fibrosis – has a better prognosis than UIP as it responds to steroids.
- MRI scan is useful in determining disease activity without ionising radiation but it is an expensive method.

Mention some prognostic factors.

Short duration of disease, young age of patient at onset, and presence of little fibrosis on lung biopsies are good prognostic factors.

How would you manage this patient?

- All patients except the elderly should receive a course of steroids: prednisolone 40 mg per day for 6 weeks. Monitor symptoms, CXR, lung function tests. If response is good, continue; if no response then taper over 1 week.
- Steroid nonresponders may benefit from a course of cyclophosphamide.
- Identify the underlying cause and manage accordingly.

What is the prognosis?

The 5-year overall survival is 50%, 65% in steroid responders and 25% in steroid nonresponders.

What are the causes of death in such patients?

- Respiratory failure or cor pulmonale precipitated by chest infections.
- 10-fold increase in bronchogenic carcinoma as compared to normal controls.

What do you know about the Hamman–Rich syndrome?

The Hamman–Rich syndrome is a rapidly progressive and fatal variant of interstitial lung disease described by Hamman and Rich.

LV Hamman (1877–1946), physician, and AR Rich (1893–1968), pathologist, worked at the Johns Hopkins Hospitals, Baltimore.
Dame Margret Turner-Warwick, contemporary chest physician, was the first woman President of the Royal College of Physicians of London; her chief interest is fibrotic lung disease.

References

Fulmer, JD (1982) An introduction to the interstitial lung disease. *Clin Chest Med* **3**: 457.

Hamman, L & Rich, AR (1944) Acute diffuse interstitial fibrosis of the lungs. *Bull Johns Hopkins Hosps* **74**: 177.

McFadden, RG, Carr, TJ & Wood TE (1987) Proton magnetic resonance imaging to stage activity of interstitial lung disease. *Chest* **92**: 31.

Tenholder, MF, Russel, MD, Knight, E et al (1987) Orthodexia. A new finding in interstitial fibrosis. *Am Rev Respir Dis* **136**: 170.

Turner-Warwick, M & Haslam, PL (1987) The value of serial bronchoalveolar lavages in assessing the clinical progress of patients with cryptogenic fibrosing alveolitis. *Am Rev Respir Dis* **135**: 26.

Turner-Warwick, M, Lebowitz, M, Burows, B & Johnson, A (1980) Cryptogenic fibrosing alveolitis and lung cancer. *Thorax* **35**: 496.

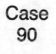 ## Case 90   Pulmonary Fibrosis

Instruction

Examine this patient's chest.

Salient features

- The fibrosis is usually apical.
- Flattening of the chest on the affected side.
- Tracheal deviation to the affected side.
- Reduced expansion on the affected side.
- Dull percussion note.
- Presence of localised crackles and bronchial breathing may be present.

- Look for the following signs:
    Scars of phrenic nerve crush, plombage, thoracotomy.
    Radiation scars.

Questions

Mention a few causes of upper lobe fibrosis.

- Tuberculosis.

- Ankylosing spondylitis.
- Radiation-induced fibrosis.

| Case 91 | Pneumothorax |

Instruction

Examine this patient's chest.

Salient features

- Decreased movement of affected side.
- Trachea may be central (small pneumothorax) or deviated to the affected side (underlying collapse of lung) or to the opposite side (large pneumothorax).
- Increased vocal resonance with diminished breath sounds.

- Look for clues regarding aetiology:
    Pleural aspiration site.
    Infraclavicular region for bruise of central line.
    Comment if the patient is a thin man or has Marfanoid features.
- Tell the examiner that you would like to take a history of wheeze (bronchial asthma, COAD).

Questions

What do you understand by the term 'pneumothorax'?

Air in the pleural cavity.

How would you investigate this patient?

- CXR, both inspiratory and expiratory.
- Blood gases if the patient is breathless.

How would you manage this patient?

- Small pneumothoraces (less than 20% in size) spontaneously resolve within weeks.
- Larger ones are managed by underwater seal drainage, which should be left in for at least 24 hours. When the lung re-expands clamp the tube for 24 hours. If a repeat CXR shows that the lung remains expanded, the tube can be removed. If not, suction should be applied to the tube. If it fails to resolve within a week, surgical pleurodesis should be considered.

What are the causes of a pneumothorax?

- Spontaneous (usually in thin males).
- Trauma.
- Bronchial asthma.
- COAD – emphysematous bulla.
- Carcinoma of the lung.
- Cystic fibrosis.
- TB.
- Mechanical ventilation.
- Marfan's syndrome, Ehlers–Danlos syndrome.
- Catamenial pneumothorax, i.e. pneumothorax which occurs in association with menstruation.

■ How would you do a pleurodesis?

By injecting talc into the pleural cavity through the intercostal tube.

In which patients would you not do a pleurodesis?

In patients with underlying cystic fibrosis. These patients may require a lung transplantation in the future and this procedure is not feasible if a pleurodesis has been carried out.

When would you suspect a tension pneumothorax?

Tension pneumothorax should be suspected in the presence of any of the following:
    Severely progressive dyspnoea.
    Severe tachycardia.
    Hypotension.
    Marked mediastinal shift.

When should open thoracotomy be considered?

It should be considered if there is one of the following present:
    A third episode of spontaneous pneumothorax.
    Any occurrence of bilateral pneumothorax.

Failure of the lung to expand after tube thoracostomy for the first episode.

OK Williamson (1866–1941), an English physician, described the Williamson sign, i.e. blood pressure in the leg is lower than that in the upper limb on the affected side in a pnuemothorax.

References

Miller, KS & Sahn, SA (1987) Chest tubes: indications, techniques, management and complications. *Chest* **91**: 258.

| Case 92 | Old Tuberculosis |

Instruction

Examine this patient's chest.

Salient features

These patients tend to have signs of the common chest cases which are not cut and dried. There are several reasons for this, such as pleural thickening, thoracotomy and pneumonectomy, associated COAD, associated chest infection, plombage or phrenic nerve crush.
   Following are some examples.

Patient 1

The candidate was asked to examine the chest from the front, as a result of which the old thoracotomy scar was not seen. The patient was wheezy. Trachea was deviated to the right. Percussion note was stony dull from the right second intercostal space downwards. Wheeze was present on the left side: this patient had a right pneumonectomy with COAD in his left lung. The candidate's diagnosis of right-sided pleural effusion with underlying collapse and left-sided COAD was accepted.

Patient 2

Trachea was central. Phrenic nerve crush scar was seen. Percussion note was dull in the left infra-axillary region and there were underlying crackles. The diagnosis of pleural thickening with associated chest infection was accepted. The diagnosis of pleural effusion was not accepted.

Questions

How would you manage a patient with old tuberculosis?

Old tuberculosis requires no antituberculosis treatment. However, the patient may require symptomatic treatment for wheeze and shortness of breath.

In which groups of patients is the risk of tuberculosis high?

- Asian and Irish immigrants.
- The elderly.
- Immunocompromised individuals, particularly AIDS patients.
- Alcoholics.
- Occupations at risk: doctors, nurses, chest physiotherapists.

■ Would you isolate a newly diagnosed, sputum-positive, pulmonary TB?

Yes. Segregation in a single room for two weeks is recommended for patients with smear-positive tuberculosis. Barrier nursing, however, is unnecessary. Adults with smear-negative or nonpulmonary disease may be in a general ward. A child with TB should be segregated until the source case is identified as this person may be visiting the child.

How are contacts investigated?

Contacts are investigated by inquiry into bacille Calmette–Guérin (BCG) vaccination state, Heaf testing and CXR examination.

To whom would you offer BCG vaccination?

BCG vaccination is offered to previously unvaccinated, persistently Heaf-test-negative or grade 1 contacts aged under 35 but not to those over 35 unless there is a special occupational, travel or ethnic risk.

What are the indications for chemoprophylaxis?

- Chemoprophylaxis may be given to those with strongly positive Heaf test reactions but no clinical or radiological evidence of TB.
- Chemoprophylaxis should be given to children under 5 who are close contacts of a smear-positive adult irrespective of their tuberculin state.
- If chemoprophylaxis is not undertaken, follow-up with periodic CXR examinations for 2 years is recommended in all these groups.

References

British Thoracic Society (1990) Control and prevention of tuberculosis in Britain: an updated code of practice. *Br Med J* **300:** 995.

Case 93 | Pickwickian Syndrome

Instruction

Look at this patient.

Salient features

- Obese patient who is plethoric and cyanosed.
- Short of breath at rest.
- May be nodding off to sleep.

- Looks for signs of pulmonary hypertension and right heart failure.
- Tell the examiner that you would like to take a history of the following:
    Snoring.
    Daytime somnolence.
    Headache.
    Poor concentration.

Questions

What is the cause of cyanosis in such a patient?

A mixture of obstructive apnoea and sleep-induced hypoventilation. The blood gas picture is hypoxia with carbon dioxide retention.

Where is the obstruction?

It is caused by the apposition of the tongue and the palate of the posterior pharyngeal wall.

How would you treat such patients?

- Weight reduction.
- Avoidance of smoking and alcohol.
- Progesterone (enhances respiratory drive).
- Continuous nasal positive airway pressure delivered by a nasal mask.

Mr Pickwick is a character in the novel *Pickwick Papers*, written by Charles Dickens, and this term was first applied by Sir William Osler.

ABDOMEN

Examination of the Abdomen

1. Ensure the patient is lying flat (remove any extra pillows, if present, with the permission of the patient) and the hands should lie by his or her side with the abdomen exposed from the infra-mammary region to just above the genitalia. Do not expose the genitalia.

2. Begin with the hands, looking for the following signs:
   - Clubbing, leuconychia (white chalky nails),
   - Palmar erythema.
   - Dupuytren's contracture (feel for thickening of the fascia).
   - Hepatic flap.

3. Examine the arms:
   - Look for arteriovenous fistulas, haemodialysis, spider naevi.

4. Comment on the skin:
   - Pigmentation.
   - Scratch marks.

5. Examine the following:
   - Supraclavicular and cervical lymph nodes.
   - Tongue for pallor.
   - Eyes for anaemia, jaundice, xanthelasma.
   - Upper chest and face for spider naevi.
   - Axilla for hair loss, acanthosis nigricans.
   - Breasts for gynaecomastia.

6. Inspect the abdomen, looking for the following signs:
   - Movements.
   - Any obvious fullness or mass.
   - Visible veins (check direction of flow which is usually away from the umbilicus).
   - Visible peristalsis.

- Hernial orifices (ask the patient to cough at this stage).
- Expansile pulsation of aortic aneurysm.

7. Ask the patient if his or her abdomen is sore in any part.

8. Palpation. Kneel on the floor or sit on a chair before you begin palpation. At all times look at the patient's eyes to check whether he or she winces for pain. Begin with superficial palpation and begin in the least tender area. Palpate in all the quadrants (remember that there are four quadrants!).

9. Palpate:
   - For mass – determine its characteristics.
   - Liver (percuss for upper border using heavy percussion, for lower border using light percussion).
   - Spleen (percuss to confirm your palpatory findings).
   - Kidneys (bimanual palpation, demonstrate ballottement).
   - Groin for lymph nodes.
   - Check hernial orifices.
   - Test for expansile pulsation of an aortic aneurysm.

10. Percuss, looking for shifting dullness (at this stage, when the patient is lying on his or her right side, seize the opportunity to examine for a small spleen and for pitting oedema over the sacral region). Remember that abdominal percussion should follow adequate inspection and palpation.

11. Auscultate:
    - Over an enlarged liver for bruit.
    - Over a suspected aortic aneurysm.
    - For bowel sounds.

12. Tell the examiner that you would like to perform a rectal examination and examine the external genitalia.

13. Examine the legs for oedema.

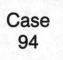

Case 94 Hepatomegaly

Instruction

Examine this patient's abdomen.

Salient features

- Enlarged liver: comment on its size, tenderness, surface (smooth or irregular); percuss the upper border (normally in the fifth intercostal space in the right midclavicular line) and auscultate for bruit.
- Look for the following signs:
  Spleen, ascites.
  Signs of cirrhosis.
  Lymph nodes.
  Raised JVP.
- At this stage you may be asked to look for nervous system signs of alcoholism (peripheral neuropathy, proximal myopathy, cerebellar syndrome, bilateral sixth cranial nerve palsy as in Wernicke's encephalopathy, recent memory loss and confabulation in Korsakoff's psychosis).

Questions

What does a tender liver indicate?

A stretch of its capsule due to a *recent* enlargement, as in cardiac failure or acute hepatitis.

What are the common causes of a palpable liver in the UK?

- Cardiac failure.
- Cirrhosis.
- Secondaries in the liver.

Mention some less common causes of hepatomegaly.

- Leukaemia and other reticuloendothelial disorders.
- Infections – glandular fever, infectious hepatitis.

- Primary biliary cirrhosis.
- Haemochromatosis.
- Sarcoid, amyloid.
- Tumours – hepatoma, hydatid cysts.

In which condition does a pulsatile liver occur?

Tricuspid regurgitation.

What does a bruit over the liver indicate?

An underlying hepatoma.

Dame Sheila Sherlock, Emeritus Professor of Medicine, Royal Free Hospital, London, is a doyen of liver diseases.
HO Thomas, contemporary Professor of Medicine, St Mary's Hospital, London; his main interest is viral hepatitis.

References

Sherlock, S (1989) *Diseases of the Liver and Biliary System* 8th edn. Oxford: Blackwell Scientific Publications.

Case 95   Cirrhosis of the Liver

Instruction

Examine this patient's abdomen.

Salient features

- In the hands:
    Clubbing, leuconychia.
    Dupuytren's contracture, palmar erythema.

Spider naevi, tattoos, hepatic flap, pallor.
Scratch marks, generalised pigmentation.
- Eyes and face:
  Icterus, cyanosis, parotid enlargement.
- Chest:
  Spider naevi, loss of axillary hair, gynaecomastia.
- Abdomen:
  Splenomegaly (seldom more than 5 cm below the costal margin).
  Ascites.
  Hepatomegaly (particularly in alcoholic liver disease).
- Pedal oedema.

Questions

What is your diagnosis?

Cirrhosis with portal hypertension due to:

- Alcohol dependence.
- Hepatitis B virus infection (look for tattoos).
- Lupoid hepatitis.
- Primary biliary cirrhosis.
- Haemochromatosis.
- Drugs – methyldopa, amiodarone, methotrexate.
- Metabolic: Wilson's disease, α_1-antitrypsin deficiency.
- Cryptogenic.

How would you investigate this patient?

- FBC including haemoglobin, platelet count.
- Liver function tests including γ-glutamyl transpeptidase (γ-GT).
- Prothrombin time.
- Hepatitis B markers.
- Serum autoantibodies.
- Serum iron and ferritin.
- Serum α-fetoprotein.
- Ascitic fluid analysis.
- Ultrasound of liver.
- Technetium isotope scan of liver.

Why does this patient have a low serum albumin concentration?

Albumin is synthesised in the liver and in cirrhosis there is liver cell failure, causing diminished synthesis.

What are the major sequelae of cirrhosis?

- Portal hypertension.
- Variceal haemorrhages.
- Hepatic encephalopathy.
- Ascites and spontaneous bacterial peritonitis.
- Hepatorenal syndrome.
- Coagulopathy.
- Hepatocellular carcinoma.

What is cirrhosis?

Cirrhosis is defined pathologically as a diffuse liver abnormality characterised by fibrosis and abnormal regenerating nodules.

What are the poor prognostic factors?

- Encephalopathy.
- Low sodium, less than $120 \, \text{mmol} \, l^{-1}$ (not due to diuretic therapy).
- Low albumin, less than $25 \, \text{g} \, l^{-1}$.
- Prolonged prothrombin time.

What factors can precipitate hepatic encephalopathy in a patient with previously well-compensated hepatic cirrhosis?

- Infection.
- Diuretics, electrolyte imbalance.
- Diarrhoea and vomiting.
- Sedatives.
- Upper gastrointestinal haemorrhage.
- Abdominal paracentesis.
- Surgery.

Case 96	Jaundice

Instruction

Would you like to ask this patient (*Patient 1*) a few questions?

Salient features

* Ask the patient about the following:
  His or her age (hepatitis is more common in the young and carcinoma in the elderly).
  Occupation (Weil's disease in sewerage and farm workers).
  Contact with jaundice (hepatitis A).
  Drug history (oral contraceptives, phenothiazines).
  Blood transfusions, injections (hepatitis B).
  Alcohol consumption.
  Colour of urine.
  Colour of stools (pale stools in obstructive jaundice).
  Abdominal pain (cholecystitis, gallstones, cholangitis, carcinoma of the pancreas).
  Family history (Gilbert's syndrome).
  Past history (recurrent jaundice, as in Dubin–Johnson syndrome).

Instruction

Would you like to examine this icteric patient (*Patient 2*)?

Salient features

* Examine the following:
  Hands (clubbing, palmar erythema, Dupuytren's contracture).
  Sclera (to confirm the icterus).
  Conjunctiva (for pallor).
  Neck (lymph nodes).
  Upper chest (spider naevi, loss of axillary hair and gynaecomastia).

Abdomen (hepatomegaly, splenomegaly, Murphy's sign, palpable gall bladder, ascites).
Legs (for pitting oedema).
• Tell the examiner that you would like to investigate as follows:
Examine the urine.
Do a per rectal examination.

Questions

What is Murphy's sign and what does it indicate?

It is the tenderness elicited on palpation at the midpoint of the right subcostal margin on inspiration. It is a sign of cholecystitis.

Have you heard of Courvoisier's law?

It states that in a patient with obstructive jaundice a palpable gall bladder is unlikely to be due to chronic cholecystitis.

What is Charcot's fever?

Intermittent fever associated with jaundice and abdominal discomfort in a patient with cholangitis and biliary obstruction.

How would you investigate this patient?

• Urine for bile pigments.
• FBC.
• Reticulocyte count and Coombs' test (if you suspect haemolysis).
• Liver function tests (serum albumin, bilirubin, enzymes).
• Prothrombin time.
• Viral studies (hepatitis antigen and antibodies, Epstein–Barr virus antibodies).
• Ultrasound of the abdomen (if you suspect cholestatic jaundice).
• Special investigations: mitochondrial antibodies, endoscopic retrograde choleangiopancreatography (ERCP), CT abdomen, liver biopsy.

What do you know about Dubin–Johnson syndrome?

It is a rare benign condition characterised by jaundice and pigmentation secondary to a failure of excretion of conjugated bilirubin. The liver is stained by melanin in the centrilobular zone. The bromosulphathalein test shows a late secondary rise at 90 minutes.

A Gilbert (1858–1927), Professor of Medicine at l'Hôtel Dieu in Paris.
PSA Weil (1848–1916), Professor of Medicine in Tartu, Estonia, and Berlin.

JB Murphy (1857–1916), Professor of Surgery at Northwestern University in Chicago.
J Courvoisier (1843–1918), Professor of Surgery, Basel, Switzerland.
IN Dubin, Professor of Pathology, Pennsylvania, and FB Johnson, pathologist,
Veterans Administration Hospital, Washington.

| Case 97 | Ascites |

Instruction

Examine this patient's abdomen.

Salient features

- Full flanks, and umbilicus.
- Presence of shifting dullness (always percuss with your finger parallel to the level of the fluid).

- If ascites is gross then use the 'dipping' method of palpation to feel the liver and spleen.
- Check for sacral oedema and swollen ankles.

Questions

What are causes of a distended abdomen?

Fat, fluid, faeces, flatus and fetus.

What investigations would you do to determine the underlying cause?

Diagnostic paracentesis for proteins and malignant cells, ultrasound of the abdomen, peritoneal biopsy or laparoscopy if the cause remains unclear.

What is the difference between an exudate and a transudate?

An exudate has a protein content of over $25\,g\,l^{-1}$.

What are the common causes of ascitic fluid?

- Portal hypertension with cirrhosis.
- Abdominal malignancy.
- Congestive cardiac failure.

What is the mechanism of ascites in cirrhosis?

- It is due to a combination of liver failure and portal hypertension. Liver failure decreases renal blood flow, resulting in retention of salt and water.
- Secondary hyperaldosteronism due to increased renin release and decreased metabolism of aldosterone by the liver.
- Decreased metabolism of antidiuretic hormone.
- Hypoalbuminaemia decreases colloid oncotic pressure.
- Lymphatic obstruction, resulting in a 'weeping' liver.

How would you manage ascites due to portal hypertension with cirrhosis?

- Bed rest.
- Low-sodium diet, 20 mmol per day.
- Diuretics, begin with spironolactone (aldosterone antagonist) and increase up to 400 mg per day before starting loop diuretics such as frusemide.
- Therapeutic paracentesis with infusion of salt-free albumin (reported to decrease hospital stay).
- Peritoneocaval shunts (Le Veen shunts) – limited by high rate of infection and disseminated intravascular coagulation.

What are the complications of ascites?

- Respiratory embarrassment may complicate large amount of ascites.
- Spontaneous bacterial peritonitis is seen in cirrhotics (suspected when there is an ascitic fluid leucocyte count of 500 cells per μL, or more than 250 polymorphonuclear cells per μL).

■ Mention some uncommon causes for ascitic fluid.

- Nephrotic syndrome.
- Constrictive pericarditis.
- Tuberculous peritonitis.
- Chylous ascites.
- Budd–Chiari syndrome.
- Meigs' syndrome.

What do you know about the pathogenesis of ascites in cirrhotics?

Two theories have been proposed:

- Underfilling theory: this suggests that the primary abnormality is inappropriate sequestration of fluid within the splanchnic vascular bed due to portal hypertension. This results in a decrease in intra-vascular volume and the kidney responds by retaining salt and water.
- Overflow theory: this suggests that the primary abnormality is inappropriate retention of salt and water by the kidney in the absence of volume depletion.

G Budd (1808–1882), Professor of Medicine at King's College, London.
H Chiari (1851–1916), Professor of Pathology at the German University in Prague.
JV Meigs (1892–1963), Professor of Gynaecology at Harvard, Massachusetts General Hospital.
Le Veen, gastroenterologist at the Veterans Administration Hospital in New York.

References

Crossley, JR & Williams, R (1985) Spontaneous bacterial peritonitis. *Gut* **26**: 325.
Epstein, FM (1982) Underfilling versus overfilling in hepatic ascites. *N Engl J Med* **307**: 1577.

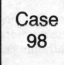

Case 98

Haemochromatosis

Instruction

Examine this patient's abdomen.
Look at this patient.

Salient features

- The patient is a pigmented male over 30 years of age.
- Palmar erythema, spider naevi.

- Jaundice.
- Ascites, hepatomegaly (firm, regular).
- Loss of secondary sexual hair.

- Tell the examiner that you would like to investigate as follows:
    Look for testicular atrophy (due to iron deposition affecting hypothalamopituitary function).
    Take a history of joint pain (present in 50% of cases): pseudogout usually affects the second and third metacarpophalangeal joints. Any of small joints may be involved.
    Examine the heart for dilated cardiomyopathy, cardiac failure.
    Check urine for sugar, looking for evidence of diabetes mellitus (present in 80% of cases).
    Remember that such patients develop cirrhosis and hepatocellular carcinoma.

Questions

Does this disease run in families?

Yes, and it is an autosomal recessive condition. It is closely associated with human leucocyte antigen HLA-A3 and to lesser extent with HLA-B14 antigen. The responsible alleles are on the short arm of chromosome 6.

Asymptomatic close relatives of patients with hereditary haemochromatosis, in particular siblings, should be advised to undergo screening tests, i.e. measurements of serum ferritin and iron, and saturation of serum iron binding capacity.

What is the benefit of early identification?

Early venesection has shown benefits, particularly in those who have not developed diabetes mellitus or cirrhosis. Early venesection prevents progression of hepatic disease and may consequently prevent complication of hepatocellular carcinoma.

How would you confirm your diagnosis?

- Transferrin saturation is increased.
- Serum ferritin levels are raised.
- Liver biopsy to measure iron stores is a definitive test.

How would you manage such a patient?

- Avoidance of alcohol.
- Venesection – weekly for 2 years (as 50 g of iron or more is deposited) and then once in 3 months.

Mention a few causes of generalised pigmentation.

Common causes are sun tan and race.
Uncommon causes are as follows:

- Liver disease: haemochromatosis in males; primary biliary cirrhosis in females.
- Addison's disease.
- Uraemia.
- Chronic debilitating conditions such as malignancy.

NDC Finlayson, contemporary gastroenterologist, Edinburgh Royal Infirmary.

References

Edwards, CQ, Griffen, LM, Goldgar, D et al (1988) Prevalence of hemochromatosis among 11065 presumably healthy blood donors. *N Engl J Med* **318:** 1355–1362.
Finlayson, NDC (1990) Hereditary (primary) haemochromatosis. *Br Med J* **309:** 351.
Niederau, C, Fischer, R, Sonnenberg, A et al (1985) Survival and causes of death in cirrhotic and in non-cirrhotic patients with primary hemochromatosis. *N Engl J Med* **313:** 1256–1262.

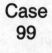

Case 99   Primary Biliary Cirrhosis

Instruction

Examine this patient's abdomen.

Salient features

- Usually occurs in middle-aged females.
- Clubbing.
- Generalised pigmentation.

- Xanthelasmata.
- Icterus.
- Scratch marks.

- Look for xanthomata over joints, skin folds and sites of trauma to the skin.
- Remember there may be clinical features of other autoimmune diseases such as rheumatoid arthritis, dry mouth of Sjögrens syndrome, systemic sclerosis, CREST syndrome (see page 224), Hashimoto's thyroiditis, dermatomyositis.
- Tell the examiner you would like to investigate as follows:
  Take history of steatorrhoea.
  Check for proximal muscle weakness due to osteomalacia.

Questions

How does primary biliary cirrhosis present?

Classically, it presents with itching in a middle-aged women. However, in 50% of cases there may be no liver symptoms.

Is there a cure for primary biliary cirrhosis?

Liver transplantation is the only known cure.

When is liver transplantation indicated?

It is indicated in those patients with liver failure and pronounced jaundice.

What drugs have been used to treat this condition?

Steriods, azathioprine, chlorambucil, cyclosporin, bile salts.

What is the rationale behind bile salt therapy?

Hepatocytes affected by autoimmune processes are further injured by endogenous bile acids (such as chenodeoxycholic acid and cholic acid) which accumulate due to associated cholestasis. Partial replacement of water-soluble bile acids such as ursodeoxycholic acid may reduce pruritus and damage to the liver cell.

Roger Williams, Professor at King's College, London and Sir Roy Calne, Professor of Surgery, Cambridge, pioneered liver transplantation in the UK.
Peter Brunt, consultant, Gastroenterology and Liver Service, Aberdeen Royal Infirmary, is also the personal physician to the Queen.

References

Bateson, MC (1990) New directions in primary biliary cirrhosis. *Br Med J* **301:** 1290.

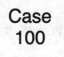

Wilson's Disease

Instruction

Look at this patient's eyes.

Salient features

- Greenish yellow to golden brown pigmentation at the limbus of the cornea, called Kayser–Fleischer ring.
- Look for the following:
  Jaundice.
  Hepatomegaly.
  Signs of liver failure.
  Sunflower cataracts.
  Neurological manifestations – tremor, chorea, masked facies.

Questions

Is Kayser–Fleischer ring pathognomonic of Wilson's disease?

No, it is also seen in primary biliary cirrhosis, chronic active hepatitis with cirrhosis, cryptogenic cirrhosis, and long-standing intrahepatic cirrhosis of childhood.

At what age do the neurological manifestations usually manifest?

They usually appear between 12 and 30 years of age. The most frequent first neurological symptom is a difficulty in speaking or writing while in school.

What are the psychiatric manifestations of this disease?

Bizarre behaviour, psychosis or hysteria.

What are the biochemical changes in Wilson's disease?

Low serum ceruloplasmin levels; serum copper may be high, low or normal; orally administered radiolabelled copper is incorporated into ceruloplasmin.

How is the diagnosis of a suspected case confirmed?

By the demonstration of one of the following:

* Kayser–Fleischer rings and a serum ceruloplasmin less than $200 \, \text{mg} \, \text{l}^{-1}$.
* A serum ceruloplasmin less than $200 \, \text{mg} \, \text{l}^{-1}$ and the concentration of copper in a liver biopsy sample greater than $250 \, \mu\text{g} \, \text{g}^{-1}$ on a dry-weight basis.

How would you treat such a patient?

Pencillamine: it removes and detoxifies deposits of copper. Treatment is lifelong and continuous.

Samuel Alexander Kinnier Wilson (1877–1937) qualified in Edinburgh and worked in Queen's Square, London, as a neurologist.
Bernhard Kayser (1869–1954) and Bruno Fleischer, both German ophthalmologists, described the same condition in 1902 and 1903 respectively.

References

Case records (44) (1984) *N Engl J Med* **311**: 1171.
Scheinberg, IH, Jaffe, ME & Sternlieb, I (1987) The use of trientine in preventing the effects of interrupting pencillamine therapy in Wilson's disease. *N Engl J Med* **317**: 209.
Wilson, SAK (1912) Progressive lenticular degeneration. A familial nervous disease associated with cirrhosis of liver. *Brain* **34**: 295.

Case 101	Splenomegaly

Instruction

Examine this patient's abdomen.

Salient features

- Massive spleen. There may be associated anaemia.
- Start low while examining for spleen and be gentle during palpation. Even if you are certain it is the spleen it is important you go through the motions of ruling out a palpable kidney: do a bimanual palpation and check for ballottement; feel for the splenic notch; auscultate for splenic rub.
- Look for enlarged lymph nodes and anaemia.
- Remember that the spleen must be at least two to three times its usual size before it is felt.
- Remember that, normally, the spleen does not extend beyond the anterior axillary line and lies along the ninth, tenth and eleventh ribs.

Questions

What is your diagnosis?

- Myeloproliferative disorder:
  Myelofibrosis, particularly in males.
  Chronic myeloid leukaemia, particularly in females.

How would you confirm your diagnosis?

Bone marrow examination.

In which other conditions is a massive spleen palpable?

- Malaria.
- Kala-azar.
- Gaucher's disease.

In which conditions is a moderately enlarged spleen (two to four finger breadths or 4–8 cm) felt?

- Portal hypertension secondary to cirrhosis.
- Lymphoproliferative disorders such as Hodgkin's disease and chronic lymphatic leukaemia.

In which common conditions would the spleen be just palpable?

- Lymphoproliferative disorders.
- Portal hypertension secondary to cirrhosis.
- Infectious hepatitis.
- Glandular fever (infectious mononucleosis).
- Subacute endocarditis.
- Sarcoid, rheumatoid arthritis, collagen disease, idiopathic thrombocytopenia, congenital spherocytosis and polycythaemia rubra vera.

PCE Gaucher (1854–1918), Professor of Dermatology in France.
Sir David Weatherall, FRS, contemporary Regius Professor of Medicine, Oxford, who has the unique distinction of being both a molecular biologist and an astute clinician.

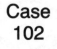

Case 102   Felty's Syndrome

Instruction

Examine this patient's abdomen.

Salient features

- Mild to moderate splenomegaly.
- Rheumatoid arthritis.

- Look for the following signs:
  Anaemia.
  Vasculitis.
  Diffuse pigmentation.
  Leg ulcers.

Questions

What is Felty's syndrome?

It is a rare complication of rheumatoid arthritis in which there is leucopenia with selective neutropenia and splenomegaly. The prognosis is poor because of recurrent Gram-positive infections.

Note. Splenectomy does not prevent sepsis.

What do you understand by the term 'hypersplenism'?

It implies removal of erythrocytes, granulocytes or platelets from the circulation by the spleen. Removal of the spleen is indicated when the underlying disorder cannot be corrected.
  Criteria for hypersplenism include the following:

- Enlarged spleen.
- Destruction of one or more cell lines in the spleen.
- Normal bone marrow.

Augustus R Felty (1895–1964) was a physician at Hartford Hospital, Hartford, Connecticut. He described this syndrome while he was working at the Johns Hopkins Hospital, Baltimore.

References

Thorne, C & Urowitz, MB (1982) Long-term outcome in Felty's syndrome. *Ann Rheum Dis* **41:** 486.

| Case 103 | Polycystic Kidneys |

Instruction

Examine this patient's abdomen.

Salient features

- Arteriovenous fistulas in the arms or subclavian dialysis catheter (remember that polycystic kidneys constitute the third commonest cause for chronic renal failure in the UK after glomerulonephritis and pyelonephritis).
- Palpable kidneys (confirm by bimanual palpation and ballottement; there is a resonant note on percussion due to over-lying colon; the hand can get between swelling and the costal margin).

- Look for the following signs:
  Enlarged liver due to cystic disease.
  Transplanted kidney may be palpable in either iliac fossa.
  Third nerve palsy (berry aneurysms are associated with polycystic kidneys).
  Bruits from intravascular anomalies (auscultate over the eyes).
- Tell the examiner you would like to investigate as follows:
  Check the blood pressure (hypertension develops in 75% of cases).
  Take a family history.
  Look for anaemia (due to chronic renal failure) or polycythaemia (due to increased erythropoiesis).
  Microscopic haematuria.

Questions

How may polycystic kidneys present?

Haematuria, hypertension, urinary tract infection, pain in the lumbar region, uraemic symptoms.

How would you like to manage this patient?

- FBC, U&E, serum creatinine, urine microscopy, urine culture.
- Ultrasound of the kidneys to confirm the diagnosis.
- Family should be screened (since it is autosomal dominant with nearly 100% penetrance).

In which other organs are cysts seen in this condition?

Liver (in 30% of cases), spleen, pancreas, lungs, ovaries, testes, epididymis, thyroid, uterus, broad ligament and bladder.

What are the neurological manifestations of this condition?

Subarachnoid haemorrhage from an intracranial berry aneurysm which causes death or neurological lesions in about 9% of patients.

■ What is the pathology?

Cysts develop in the Bowman's capsule and at other levels in the nephron, displacing kidney tissue.

What cardiovascular manifestations have been reported in these patients?

- Mitral valve prolapse in 26%.
- Other lesions commonly seen are mitral, aortic and tricuspid valve regurgitation.

What do you know about the genetic transmission of this disease?

The inheritance is autosomal dominant and in most families it is linked to the α-haemoglobin gene complex and the phosphoglycerate kinase genes at the PKD 1 locus on the short arm of the chromosome 16. However, in 4% of families with the disorder it is caused by unknown mutations elsewhere in the genome.

Sir W Bowman (1816–1892), surgeon at the Royal London Ophthalmic Hospital.
Jerome Kassirer, renal physician and Editor-in-Chief of the *New England Journal of Medicine*.

References

Chauveau, D, Sirieix, M, Schillinger, F, Legendre, C & Grunfeld, J (1990) Recurrent rupture of intracranial aneurysms in autosomal dominant polycystic kidney disease. *Br Med J* **301**: 966–967.

DeBono, DP & Evans, DB (1977) The management of polycystic kidney disease with special reference to dialysis and transplantation. *Q J Med* **183**: 63–66.

Kimberling, WF, Fain, PR, Kenyon, JB et al (1988) Linkage heterogeneity of autosomal dominant polycystic kidney disease. *N Engl J Med* **319**: 913.

Levey, AS, Panker, SG & Kassirer, JP (1983) Occult intracranial aneurysms in polycystic kidney disease. When is cerebral arteriography warranted? *N Engl J Med* **308**: 986–994.

Case 104	Unilateral Palpable Kidney

Instruction

Examine this patient's abdomen.

Salient features

- One kidney is palpable (bimanually ballottable; there is a transverse band of colonic resonance on percussion and you will be able to insinuate your fingers bctween the mass and costal margin).

- Look carefully for arteriovenous fistulas in the arms, haemodialysis catheters in the subclavian region.

Questions

What are the common causes for a palpable kidney?

- Polycystic kidney disease.
- Carcinoma.
- Hydronephrosis.
- Renal cyst.
- Hypertrophy of solitary functioning kidney.

What changes can occur in a kidney when the other is removed?

Long-term renal function remains stable in most patients with a reduction in renal mass of more than 50%. However, these patients are at increased risk for proteinuria, glomerulopathy and progressive renal failure. Hence it is important to monitor patients with remnant kidneys. Problems are most frequent in those in whom the amount of renal tissue removed is greatest and who have survived the longest.

Graeme Catto, contemporary Professor of Renal Medicine and Dean, Aberdeen Medical School is a keen proponent of the NHS reform and trust status.
Leon Fine, contemporary Professor of Medicine, University College Hospital, London.
HA Lee, contemporary Professor of Renal Medicine, Portsmouth, is also interested in metabolism.

References

Fine, LG (1991) How little kidney tissue is enough? *N Engl J Med* 325: 1097.
Novick, AC, Gephardt, G, Guz, B, Steinmuller, D & Tubbs, RR (1991) Long term follow up after partial removal of a solitary kidney. *N Engl J Med* 325: 1058.

Case 105 Abdominal Masses

Instruction

Examine this patient's abdomen.

Salient features

Patient 1 has an epigastric mass. Differential diagnosis:

* Carcinoma of the stomach: look for supraclavicular lymph nodes, hepatomegaly; comment on pallor and asthenia.
* Carcinoma of the pancreas: look for jaundice.

- Aneurysm of the abdominal aorta: look for pulsatile mass; check femoral and foot pulses; auscultate over the mass and the femoral pulses.
- Retroperitoneal lymphadenopathy (lymphoma).

Patient 2 has a mass in the right iliac fossa. Differential diagnosis:

- Crohn's disease: look for mouth ulcers; tell the examiner that you would like to look for fistulas and take a history of chronic diarrhoea.
- Carcinoma of the caecum: look for hard mass, lymph nodes.
- Look for lymph nodes elsewhere (see page 326); feel for liver and spleen; examine the drainage area of iliac lymph nodes (such as the leg, perianal area, external genitalia; do a rectal examination).
- Transplanted kidney: comment on the laparotomy scars, stigmata of renal failure and artificial arteriovenous fistulas.
- Appendicular abscess.
- Ileocaecal abscess, particularly in Asians.
- Ovarian tumours (must be mentioned as a differential diagnosis in female patients).

Less common causes of mass in the right iliac fossa:

- Amoebiasis.
- Carcinoid (ileal).
- Actinomycosis.
- Ectopic kidney.

Patient 3 has a mass in the left iliac fossa. Differential diagnosis:

- Diverticular abscess: look for tender, mobile mass.
- Carcinoma colon: look for hepatomegaly; tell the examiner that you would like to do a per rectal examination.
- Faecal mass (the mass may be moulded by pressure).
- Ovarian tumour (in females).
- Iliac lymph nodes: look for other lymph nodes, liver and spleen; examine the drainage areas.
- Transplanted kidney: comment on the laparotomy scar; look for signs of renal failure, arteriovenous fistulas.

Note. The investigation of first choice in such patients is an abdominal ultrasound.

RHEUMATOLOGY

Examination of the Hands

1. Ask the patient, 'Are your hands painful?'.

2. Inspect for joint deformity:
   - Swan-neck deformity (flexion at the distal interphalangeal joints and hyperextension of the proximal interphalangeal joints).
   - Boutonnière deformity (flexion of proximal interphalangeal joints and hyperextension of the distal interphalangeal joint).
   - Z deformity of the thumb.
   - Ulnar deviation of the fingers.

3. Examine the nails:
   - Nail fold infarcts (rheumatoid arthritis).
   - Nail pitting, onycholysis, ridging, hyperkeratosis, discoloration (psoriasis).

4. Comment on the following:
   - Wasting of the small muscles of the hands, in particular those on the dorsum of the hand.
   - Heberden's nodes, i.e. bony nodules at the distal interphalangeal joints (osteoarthroses).
   - Bouchard's nodes, i.e. bony nodules at the proximal interphalangeal joints (osteoarthroses).
   - Spindle-shaped deformity of the fingers.
   - Gouty tophi.

5. Examine the palms:
   - Wasting of the thenar or hypothenar eminence.
   - Thickening of the palmar fascia – Dupuytren's contracture (rheumatoid arthritis).
   - Palmar erythema (rheumatoid arthritis).
   - Tap over the flexor retinaculum to detect median nerve entrapment (Tinel's sign).

6. Get the patient to perform the following movements:
   - Unbuttoning of clothes.
   - Pincer movements.
   - Hand grip.
   - Abduction of the thumb.
   - Writing.

7. Test sensation of the index and little fingers.

8. Examine the elbows for the following signs:
   - Rheumatoid nodules.
   - Gouty tophi.
   - Psoriatic plaques.

9. Tell the examiner that you would like to examine the other joints.

Note. When asked to examine the hands consider the possibilities of arthropathy, myopathy, neuropathy, a peripheral nerve lesion or acromegaly.

W Heberden, Sr (1710–1801), English physician.
CJ Bouchard (1837–1915), French physician.

General Guidelines for Examination of Joints

History

Ask the patient if he or she has any pain, stiffness, or difficulty in dressing or walking.

Examination

- *Look* at posture, gait and joint deformity.
- *Feel* for temperature, tenderness, joint fluid and crepitus of movement of the joints.
- *Move*: check passive and active movements of the joints; test stability of the joints.
- *Measure* muscle wasting and shortening of the limb.

Examination of the knees:

- Ask the patient if the joints are sore.
- Expose both knees and lower thighs fully with the patient lying supine.

- Look for:
  Quadriceps wasting.
  Swelling of the joint.
- Feel:
  Temperature.
  Synovial thickening.
  Do the patellar tap (ballottement): the fluid from the supra-patellar bursa is forced into the joint space by squeezing the lower part of the quadcriceps and then the patellar is pushed posteriorly with the fingers; this test indicates fluid in the synovial cavity.
- Movement:
  Test passive flexion and extension – make a note of the range of movement and feel for crepitus.
  Gently extend the knee and examine for fixed flexion deformity.
  Test the medial and lateral ligaments by steadying the thigh with the left hand and moving the leg with the right laterally and medi-ally when the knee joint is slightly flexed – movements more than 10 degrees are abnormal.
  Test the cruciate ligaments by steadying the foot with your elbow and moving the leg anteriorly and posteriorly with the other hand – laxity more than 10 degrees is abnormal.
- Ask the patient to lie on his or her stomach and feel the popliteal fossa when the knee is extended.

Examination of the feet:

- Look:
  For skin rash, scars.
  At the nails for changes of psoriasis.
  At the forefoot for hallux valgus, clawing and crowding of the toes (rheumatoid arthritis).
  At the callus over the metatarsal heads which may occur in subluxation.
  At both the arches of the foot, in particular medial and longitud-inal (flat foot, pes cavus).
- Palpate:
  The ankles, for synovitis, effusion, passive movements at the subtalar joint (inversion and eversion) and talar joint (dorsiflex-ion and plantar flexion); remember that tenderness on movement is more important than the range of movement
  Metatarsophalangeal joints, for tenderness.
  The individual digits, for synovial thickening.
  The bottom of the heel, for tenderness (plantar fasciitis), and the Achilles tendon for nodules.

Case 106	Rheumatoid Hands

Instruction

Examine this patient's hands.

Salient features

- Ask the patient for permission to examine his or her hands and then ask if the hands are sore.
- Comment on deformities such as the following:
  Subluxation at the metacarpophalangeal joint.
  Swan-neck deformity.
  Boutonnière deformity (hyperextension at the terminal interphalangeal joint and flexion at the proximal interphalangeal joint).
  Z deformity of the thumb.
  Dorsal subluxation of ulna at the carpal joint.
- Comment on the following signs:
  Nail fold infarcts and vasculitic skin lesions.
  Palmar erythema.
  Wasting of the first dorsal interossei and other small muscles of the hand.
- Test grip and pincer movements. Quickly test for abductor pollicis brevis and interossei, and pinprick sensation over index and little fingers. The median nerve may be involved if there is an associated carpal tunnel syndrome.
- Examine the elbow for rheumatoid nodules.
- Ask the patient to perform simple tasks involving hand function, such as unbuttoning his or her clothes, or writing.
- Tell the examiner that you would like to examine other joints.
- Highlight the following points:
  Whether terminal interphalangeal joints are spared or affected.
  Whether the arthritis is active (if the joints are inflamed) or inactive.

Questions

What is the significance of rheumatoid nodules?

The presence of nodules indicates seropositive and more aggressive arthritis.

Where else are nodules found?

Flexor and extensor tendons of the hand, sacrum, Achilles tendon, sclera, lungs and myocardium.

What are the skin lesions in rheumatoid arthritis?

Vasculitis, nail fold infarcts.

What are the causes of anaemia in rheumatoid arthritis?

- Anaemia of chronic disease.
- Megaloblastic anaemia due to folate deficiency or associated pernicious anaemia.
- Felty's syndrome.
- Drugs: nonsteroidal anti-inflammatory drugs (NSAIDs) causing iron deficiency anaemia; bone marrow suppression caused by gold.

What is Felty's syndrome (see page 204)?

It is seen in some patients with severe rheumatoid arthritis and consists of splenomegaly, anaemia, leucopenia and thrombocytopenia (hypersplenism), and leg ulcers. Splenectomy ameliorates hypersplenism. Felty's syndrome is associated with positive rheumatoid factor.

What are the pulmonary manifestations of rheumatoid arthritis?

- Pleural effusion or pleurisy (seen in 25% of men with rheumatoid arthritis).
- Rheumatoid nodules.
- Fibrosing alveolitis.
- Caplan's syndrome (rheumatoid arthritis coexists with rounded fibrotic nodules 0.5–5 cm in diameter mainly in the periphery of lung fields in coal-worker's pneumoconiosis).

What are the eye manifestations of rheumatoid arthritis?

- Episcleritis.
- Scleritis.
- Scleromalacia, scleromalacia perforans.
- Keratoconjuctivitis sicca.
- Sjögren's syndrome (see above).

What precautions are necessary before upper gastrointestinal endoscopy or general anaesthesia?

It is prudent to take a cervical spine X-ray in order to rule out atlantoaxial subluxation.

Which joints are commonly affected in rheumatoid arthritis?

Wrists, proximal interphalangeal joints and metacarpophalangeal joints of hands, metatarsophalangeal joints, knees.

What is palindromic rheumatoid arthritis?

Palindromic onset is seen in some patients with recurrent episodes of joint stiffness and pain in individual joints lasting only a few hours or days. Hydroxychloroquine may be of value in preventing recurrences.

■ How would you treat the arthritis?

Prescribe NSAIDs including aspirin. If, after a month of NSAID, the symptoms persist with no sign of remission then a second line drug should be added. Second line drugs include hydroxychloroquine, sulphasalazine and pencillamine. Low-dose methotrexate and gold salts are also used to prevent disease progression.

If the patient is known to experience gastric distress with NSAIDs then what precautions would you take while prescribing them?

Prophylaxis for NSAID-associated gastric distress may be attempted with concurrent administration of an H_2 blocker such as ranitidine, omeprazole or misoprostol. The latter is a prostaglandin analogue which is reputed to protect the mucosa.

What are the neurological manifestations of rheumatoid arthritis?

- Peripheral neuropathy – glove and stocking sensory loss.
- Mononeuritis multiplex.
- Entrapment neuropathy, e.g. carpal tunnel syndrome.
- Cervical disease or atlantoaxial subluxation may cause cervical myelopathy.

What are the causes of proteinuria in patients with rheumatoid arthritis?

- Drug therapy: gold salts, pencillamine.
- Amyloidosis.

What is Sjögren's syndrome?

The association of keratoconjuctivitis sicca (lack of lacrimal secretion) and xerostomia (dry mouth due to lack of salivary gland secretion) in association with a connective tissue disorder, usually rheumatoid arthritis. This syndrome may also be associated with autoimmune thyroid disease, myasthenia gravis or autoimmune liver disease.

- The Schirmer filter paper test provides a crude measure of tear production. Filter paper is hooked over the lower eyelid and in normal people at least 15 mm is wet after 5 minutes whereas in sicca syndrome it is less than 5 mm.
- Anti-Ro (SSA) and anti-SS-B antibodies may be seen in this syndrome.
- Treatment is symptomatic with artificial tears (hypomellose drops or 1% methylcellulose), artificial saliva and NSAIDs for the arthritis.

What are the criteria for rheumatoid arthritis?

American Rheumatism Association criteria:

1. Morning stiffness for at least 1 hour for a duration of 6 weeks or more.
2. Swelling of at least three joints for 6 weeks or more.
3. Swelling of wrist, metacarpophalangeal or proximal interphalangeal joints for 6 weeks or more.
4. Symmetry of swollen joint areas for 6 weeks or more.
5. Subcutaneous nodules.
6. Positive rheumatoid factor.
7. X-ray features typical of rheumatoid arthritis, i.e. erosions and periarticular osteopenia.

When four or more of the above criteria are met they show 93% sensitivity and 90% specificity. It is important to note that the diagnosis of rheumatoid arthritis should not be made on the basis of these criteria alone if another systemic disease associated with arthritis is definitely present.

What are poor prognostic factors?

- Systemic features: weight loss, extra-articular manifestations.
- Insidious onset.
- Rheumatoid nodules.
- Presence of rheumatoid factor more than 1 in 512.
- Persistent activity of the disease for over 12 months.
- Early bone erosions.

What are the factors leading to ulnar deviation of the hands?

- In the normal grip the fingers move into ulnar deviation.

- Weakening of radial sides of the joint capsule and radial insertion of the interossei ligaments.
- The volar supports of the flexor tendon sheath are weakened by inflammation, allowing the tendon to bow in the direction of the ulna during gripping.
- Ulnar displacement of the extensor tendons in early deviation makes them slip, if the dorsal metacarpophalangeal joint is taut, and thereby exacerbate the development of ulnar deviation by acting as a bowstring.
- The joint capsules of metacarpophalangeal joints are weaker on radial sides than on ulnar sides.

HSC Sjögren was a Swedish ophthalmologist who described the condition in 1933.
A Caplan, British physician, was an industrial officer in the Welsh coal mines.

References

Arnett, FC, Edworthy, S, Bloch, DA et al (1988) The 1987 revised ARA criteria for rheumatoid arthritis. *Arthritis Rheum* **31**: 315.

Brooks, PM & Day, RO (1991) Drug therapy: nonsteroidal antiinflammatory drugs – differences and similarities. *N Engl J Med* **324**: 1716.

Graham, Y, Agrawal, NM & Roth, SH (1988) Prevention of NSAID induced gastric ulcer with misoprostol. Multicentre double, placebo controlled trial. *Lancet* **2**: 556.

Harris, ED (1990) Mechanisms of disease: rheumatoid arthritis: pathophysiology and implications for therapy. *N Engl J Med* **322**: 1277.

Wilder, RL (1988) Treatment of the patient with rheumatoid arthritis refractory to standard therapy. *JAMA* **259**: 2446.

Case 107	Ankylosing Spondylitis

Instruction

Examine this patient's back.
Examine this patient.

Salient features

- 'Question mark' posture due to loss of lumbar lordosis, fixed kyphosis of the thoracic spine with compensatory extension of the cervical spine.
- The whole body turns when the patient is asked to look to either side.
- Examine the movements of the cervical, thoracic and lumbar spines (remember that cervical spine involvement occurs later in the disease and results in pain and a grating sensation on movement of the neck).
- Comment on the protuberant abdomen.
- Examine for distal arthritis (occurs in up to 30% of patients and it may precede the onset of the back symptoms). Small joints of the hand and feet are rarely affected.
- Measure the chest expansion using a tape (less than 5 cm suggests costovertebral involvement).
- Measure the occiput-to-wall distance (inability to make contact when heel and back are against the wall indicates upper thoracic and cervical limitation).
- Tell the examiner that you would like to do the Schober's test. (This involves marking points 10 cm above and 5 cm below a line joining the 'dimple of Venus' on the sacral promontory. An increase in separation of less than 5 cm during full forward flexion indicates limited spinal mobility.)

    Note. Finger–floor distance is a simple indicator but is less reliable because good hip movement may compensate for back limitation.
- Tell the examiner that you would like to examine the following:
    Eyes for iritis, anterior uveitis (seen in 20% of patients).
    Heart for aortic regurgitation (seen in 4% of patients who have had the disease for over 15 years), cardiac conduction defects.
    Lungs for mild restrictive disease, apical fibrosis, apical cavities and secondary fungal infection.
    Central nervous system such as tetraplegia, etc.
    Foot for Achilles tendinitis and plantar fasciitis.
- Remember the four 'A's of ankylosing spondylitis: apical fibrosis, anterior uveitis, aortic regurgitation, achilles tendinitis.
- Remember that psoriasis and Reiter's syndrome can cause sacroiliitis.

Questions

What investigations would you like to do in this patient?

Anteroposterior view of sacroiliac joints and lateral X-rays of lumbar spine: the earliest changes are erosions and sclerosis of the sacroiliac joints. Later in the disease syndesmophytes may be found in the lumbosacral spine. In severe disease, involvement progresses up the spine, leading to a 'bamboo spine'.

In which other seronegative arthritis is low back pain a feature?

Sacroiliitis is often seen in Reiter's syndrome, psoriatic arthritis, juvenile chronic arthritis and intestinal arthropathy.

How would you manage a patient with ankylosing spondylitis?

- Encourage exercise, in particular physical therapy to preserve back extension.
- NSAIDs, in particular indomethacin. Phenylbutazone is reserved for resistant cases.
- Surgical therapy, consisting of a vertebral wedge osteotomy, is occasionally indicated.

■ What genetic counselling would you give this patient?

In HLA-B27-positive patients, the sibs have a 30% chance of developing this disease. Hence children of such patients who develop symptoms such as joint pains or sore eyes should be referred to a rheumatologist.

What is the natural history of this disease?

About 40% go on to develop severe spinal restriction; about 20% have significant disability, and that early peripheral joint disease, particularly of the hip, indicates a poor prognosis.

What is the risk in those with a 'bamboo' cervical spine during driving?

Increased susceptibility to whiplash injury, and restricted lateral vision.

What therapy may the patient have received in the past if his or her blood picture shows a leukaemic picture?

In the past, patients were treated with irradiation of the spine. However, such patients tend to develop leukaemia several years after therapy.

Note. The term 'ankylosing spondylitis' derives from the Greek words, *ankylos* (bent or crooked) and *spondylos* (vertebra). Past names have included Marie–Strümpell disease and von Bechterew's disease.

The first clinical report of ankylosing spondylitis (1831) concerned a man from the Isle of Man. Vladimir von Bechterew of St Petersburg, Russia, described a series of cases between 1857 and 1927. Adolf Strümpell (1853–1926), of Erlangen, and Pierre Marie (1853–1940), of Paris, independently described this condition in 1897 and 1898 respectively.

HC Reiter (1881–1969), German physician.
Achilles is a figure from Greek mythology who was a hero of the Trojan war. His mother dipped him into the Styx, holding him by his heel, to make him invulnerable to attack. He slew Hector in this war, but was himself slain, wounded in his vulnerable heel by Paris.

References

Brewerton, DA, Goddard, DH, More, RB et al (1987) The myocardium in ankylosing spondylitis. *Lancet* **1**: 995.
Carette, S, Graham, D, Little, H et al (1983) The natural disease course of ankylosing spondylitis. *Arthritis Rheum* **26**: 186.
Editorial (1971) The lungs in ankylosing spondylitis. *Br Med J* **3**: 492.
Editorial (1978) HLA B27 and the risk of ankylosing spondylitis. *Br Med J* **2**: 650–651.
Smith, RG & Doll, R. (1982) Mortality among patients with ankylosing spondylitis after a single treatment course with x-rays. *Br Med J* **284**: 449–460.

Case 108 Psoriasis

Instruction

Examine this patient's hands.

Salient features

- Distal interphalangeal joint involvement.

- Tell the examiner that you would like to investigate as follows:
  Examine the nails, looking for pitting, onycholysis, discoloration, thickening (nails are involved in 80% of those with psoriatic arthritis).
  Look for psoriatic plaques on the extensor aspects of elbows, scalp, submammary region, umbilicus and natal cleft; describe these as reddish plaques with well-defined edges and silvery white scales.

- Comment on the fingers, which are sausage shaped due to tenosynovitis.

Questions

What are the patterns of joint involvement seen in psoriasis?

- Asymmetrical terminal joint involvement.
- Symmetrical joint involvement as seen in rheumatoid arthritis.
- Sacroiliitis: this differs from ankylosing spondylitis, most notably in that the syndesmophytes tend to arise from the lateral and anterior surfaces of the vertebral bodies and not at the margins of the bodies.
- Arthritis mutilans – complicated by the 'telescoping' of digits.

What are the radiological features of psoriatic arthritis?

- 'Fluffy' periostitis.
- Destruction of small joints.
- 'Pencil and cup' appearance, osteolysis and ankylosis in arthritis mutilans.
- Nonmarginal syndesmophytes in spondylitis.

What is the prognosis?

Deforming and erosive arthritis is present in 40% of cases and 11% are disabled by their arthritis.

References

Editorial (1988) Prognosis of psoriatic arthritis. *Lancet* **2**: 375.
Lambert, JR & Wright, V (1977) Psoriatic spondylitis: a clinical and radiological description of spine in psoriatic arthritis. *Q J Med* **46**: 411.

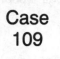

Case 109   Scleroderma

Instruction

Look at these hands.

Salient features

- Thickening and tightening of the skin over fingers, sclerodactyly (finger pulp atrophy), beaking of nails (pseudoclubbing), atrophic nails, telangiectasia (nail fold capillaries).
- Raynaud's phenomenon.
- Subcutaneous calcification (fingers, elbows and extensor aspect of forearms).
- Vitiligo or pigmentation.

- Assess hand function.
- Examine the following:
  The joints for arthralgia or arthritis.
  The face for microstomia, difficulty in opening the mouth, beak-like or pinched appearance of the nose, blotchy telangiectasia.
  The abdomen for liver (primary biliary cirrhosis).
- Tell the examiner that you would like to ask about the following:
  Dysphagia.
  Raynaud's phenomenon.
  Dry eyes.

Questions

What other organ systems are involved?

- Skin: Raynaud's phenomenon; localised morphoea; local or generalised oedema; hyperpigmentation; telangiectasia; subcutaneous calcification; ulcerations, particularly at the finger tips.
- Musculoskeletal system: arthritis; myositis; myopathy; bone ischaemia with resorption of the phalanges.
- Gastrointestinal tract: dysphagia; reflux oesophagitis; large or small bowel obstruction.
- Lung: fibrosis; atelectasis; pulmonary hypertension; pneumonia.

- Kidney: glomerulonephritis, malignant hypertension (poorest prognosis with renal involvement).
- Heart: myocardial fibrosis.

What are the variants of scleroderma?

CREST syndrome (see below), eosinophilic fasciitis, Thibierge–Weissenbach syndrome.

What is 'CREST' syndrome.

Calcinosis, Raynaud's phenomenon, oesophageal dysmotility, sclerodactyly and telangiectasia. It has a more favourable prognosis than systemic sclerosis, and is associated with the anticentromere antibody.

■ What are the criteria for diagnosis of scleroderma?

- Major criterion is proximal scleroderma (affecting metacarpophalangeals and metatarsophalangeals).
- Minor criteria are as follows:
  Sclerodactyly
  Digital tip pitting or loss of substance of distal fingers pads
  Bibasal pulmonary fibrosis.
At least the major or two or more minor criteria are required.

What are causes of anaemia in such a patient?

- Iron deficiency from chronic oesophagitis.
- Folate and vitamin B_{12} deficiency from malabsorption.
- Anaemia of chronic disease.
- Microangiopathic haemolytic anaemia.

What are the phases of skin changes in scleroderma?

- An early oedematous phase (with pitting oedema of hands and possibly forearms, legs and face).
- The dermal phase.
- An atrophic phase, followed by contracture.
- Other skin changes occur, e.g. depigmentation.

What do you know about the pathogenesis of these skin changes?

The endothelial damage resulting from a circulatory protein factor has been implicated as an early component of the 'inflammatory' phase of scleroderma and endothelial damage may result in the capillary and arteriolar abnormalities demonstrated, as well as local access of circulating proteins acting on fibroblast-enhancing collagen secretion.
Remember that the prognosis is worse in those with renal disease

and in males. Skin and/or gut involvement without other organ disease
has the best prognosis.

The first reports of scleroderma were by WD Chowne, of London, in 1842, and James
Startin, also from London, in 1846. The term 'sclerodermie' was suggested by E Gintrac
(1791–1877) of Bordeaux. Italian physician GB Fantonetti introduced the term 'sklero-
derma' in 1836.

References

Barnett, AJ, Miller, MH & Littlejohn, GD (1988) A survival study of patients with scle-
    roderma diagnosed over 30 years (1953–1983): the value of a simple cutaneous
    classification in the early stage of the disease. *J Rheumatol* 15: 276.
Lally, EV, Jimenej, SA & Kaplan, SR (1988) Progressive systemic sclerosis. Mode of
    presentation, rapidly progressive disease course and mortality based on analysis of
    91 patients. *Semin Arthritis Rheum* 118: 1.
Masi, AT, Rodnan, GP, Medsger, TA et al (1980) Preliminary criteria for classification
    of systemic sclerosis. *Arthritis Rheum* 23: 581–590.
Tumulty, PA (1968) Clinical synopsis of scleroderma, simulator of other disease. *Johns
    Hopkins Med J* 122: 236.

Case 110	Painful Knee Joint

Instruction

Examine this patient's leg.
Examine this patient's joints.
Examine this patient's knee joint.

Salient features

- Pain on movement of the joint (take care not to hurt the patient).
- Swelling of the joint (you must demonstrate fluid in the joint).

- Check both active and passive movements.
- Look for disuse atrophy of the muscles around the joint.

- Tell the examiner that you would like to investigate as follows:
  Examine other joints.
  Take a history of trauma and fever.
  X-ray the knee (anteroposterior and lateral views).
  Analyse the joint fluid for cells, sugar, protein and culture.

Questions

What are the common causes of a painful knee joint?

- Rheumatoid arthritis.
- Osteoarthrosis.
- Trauma.
- Septic arthritis (will require emergency removal of the pus to prevent joint damage).
- Viral infections.
- Gout.
- Pseudogout.
- Haemophilia.

What is palindromic rheumatoid arthritis?

Palindromic onset of rheumatoid arthritis refers to acute, recurrent arthritis usually affecting one joint with symptom-free intervals of days to months between attacks. This term was introduced by PS Hench and EF Rosenberg.

■ A patient with a painful knee joint and a unilateral facial nerve palsy is seen by you in the outpatient department. Six weeks prior to this he developed an annular rash after a camping trip in Europe. What is your diagnosis and what confirmatory test would you carry out?

The diagnosis is Lyme disease and the confirmatory test is an antibody titre against *Borrelia burgdorferi*. This disease was first recognised in Lyme, Connecticut, USA.

Case 111	Osteoarthrosis

Instruction

Look at this patient's hands.
Examine this patient's joints.

Salient features

- Heberden's nodes (bony swellings) at the terminal interphalangeal joints.
- Squaring of the hands due to subluxation of the first metacarpocarpal joint.
- Tell the examiner that you would like to examine the hips and knees as these joints are usually involved (feel the knee for crepitus: it may be red, warm and tender, and have an effusion).

Questions

Which other joints are frequently involved?

Spine, in particular cervical and lumbar spines.

Mention the types and a few causes of osteoarthrosis.

- Primary.
- Secondary:
    Trauma – affects athletes, pneumatic drill workers, anyone doing work involving heavy lifting.
    Inflammatory arthropathies – rheumatoid arthritis, septic arthritis, gout.
    Neuropathic joints – in diabetes mellitus, syringomyelia, tabes dorsalis.
    Endocrine – acromegaly, hyperparathyroidism.
    Metabolic – chondrocalcinosis, haemochromatosis.

What are Heberden's nodes?

Bony swellings seen at the terminal interphalangeal joints in osteoarthrosis.

What are Bouchard's nodes?

Bony swellings at the proximal interphalangeal joints in osteoarthrosis.

■ What are the typical radiological features?

- Subchondral bone sclerosis and cysts.
- Osteophytes.

What will synovial aspirate show?

Fewer than 100 white blood cells per millilitre.

What do you understand by the term 'nodal osteoarthrosis'?

Nodal osteoarthrosis is a primary generalised osteoarthrosis which has characteristic clinical features. It occurs predominantly in middle-aged women and is autosomal dominant. It characteristically affects the terminal interphalangeal joints with the development of Heberden's nodes. The arthritis may be acute and although there may be marked deformity there is little disability. It can also affect the carpometacarpal joints of the thumbs, spinal apophyseal joints, knees and hips.

William Heberden (1710–1801) was a London physician who described the nodes as 'little hard knobs' and this was first published posthumously in 1802.
JK Spender (1886), of Bath, introduced the term osteoarthritis. Archibald E Garrod, from London, established the modern usage and clinical differentiation from rheumatoid arthritis in 1907.
In 1884, CJ Bouchard (1837–1915) described nodes adjacent to the proximal interphalangeal joints identical to those at the distal interphalangeal joints.

References

Hamerman, D (1989) The biology of osteoarthritis. *N Engl J Med* **320:** 1322.
Moskowitz, RW (1987) Primary osteoarthritis. Epidemiology, clinical aspects and general management. *Am J Med* **83**(suppl 5A): 5.

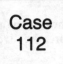

Case 112 Gout

Instruction

Examine this patient's hands or examine the feet.

Salient features

- Chronic tophaceous deposit with asymmetrical joint involvement.
- Tell the examiner that you would like to proceed as follows:
    Examine the helices of the ears, olecranon bursae and Achilles tendons for tophi.
    Examine the feet or hands.

Note. Uric acid crystals are negatively birefringent, needle shaped and may be deposited in bursae, bone and marrow. They are demonstrable in synovial fluid within leucocytes and free in the fluid during attacks of gouty arthritis. They react with nitric acid and ammonium hydroxide to give a purple colour (murexide test).

Questions

What is the basic pathophysiology of gout?

Gout is a metabolic disorder of purine metabolism. It is characterised by hyperuricaemia either due to overproduction (75%) or under-excretion (25%) of uric acid.

What are the different clinical manifestations of gout?

- Asymptomatic hyperuricaemia.
- Acute arthritis.
- Chronic arthritis.
- Chronic tophaceous gout.

How would you treat an acute attack of gout?

Prescribe an NSAID such as indomethacin. Refractory gout may require steroids.

What factors may precipitate acute gouty arthritis?

Drugs (diuretics, aspirin), copious consumption of alcohol, dehydration, surgery, fasting, foods high in purines (sweetbreads, liver, kidney, sardines).

Under what circumstances would you treat hyperuricaemia?

Frequent attacks of acute arthritis, renal damage, consistently elevated serum uric acid. Before attempting to lower serum uric acid levels it is prudent to use colchicine for preventing acute attacks.

What is the drug of choice for controlling hyperuricaemia?

Allopurinol (a xanthine oxidase inhibitor).

What drugs would you use if the patient is allergic to allopurinol?

Uricosuric drugs such as probenecid, sulphinpyrazone.

What is pseudogout?

Pseudogout is an acute arthritis resulting from the release of calcium pyrophosphate dihydrate crystals (deposited in the bone and cartilage) into the synovial fluid.

Gout has been recognised from as early as the 4th century BC. Two concepts have prevailed: that it occurs mainly in sexually mature men and that gastronomic and sexual excesses may precipitate acute attacks. Antonj van Leeuwenhoeck (1632–1723) described the microscopic appearance of urate crystals from a gouty tophus. In 1847 Alfred Garrod, in London, identified uric acid in the serum of a gouty man.

James Wyngaarden, contemporary Professor of Medicine Duke University, USA whose chief interest is metabolic and genetic diseases.

Case 113 — Ehlers–Danlos Syndrome

Instruction

Do a general examination.
Examine this patient's joints.

Salient features

Skin:

- The skin over neck, axillae and groin is smooth and elastic. It can be stretched and when released it returns immediately to its normal position. Late in the disease it becomes lax, wrinkled and hangs in folds.
- Look at bony prominences for bruising, haemotomas and gaping wounds. Wounds heal forming tissue-paper or papyraceous scars.
- Haemotomas heal forming pseudotumours or nodules.

Joints:

- Kyphoscoliosis.
- Hypermobility of the joints.

- Tell the examiner that you would like to examine the following:
    The hernial orifices.
    The heart for mitral valve prolapse and aortic regurgitation.
    The eyes for myopia, retinal detachment.

Questions

What are the gastrointestinal manifestations of this syndrome?

- Marked tendency to herniate.
- Achalasia cardia.
- Eventration of the diaphragm.
- Megacolon.

What are the cardiovascular manifestations?

- Mitral valve prolapse.
- Aortic dissection.

What are the features of hypermobility syndrome?

- Passive approximation of thumb to forearm with wrist flexion.
- Passive hyperextension of the digits.
- Active hyperextension of the knee to more than 10 degrees.
- Active hyperextension of the elbow to more than 10 degrees.
- Passive and excessive hyperextension of the foot and ankle and eversion of foot.

The diagnosis is made when any three of the above six features are present.

Edvard Ehlers (1863–1937), a Danish dermatologist, and HA Danlos, a French dermatologist, described this condition independently in 1901 and 1908 respectively.

References

Liechtenstein, JR, Martin, OR, Kohn, L, Byers, PH & McKusick, VA (1973) Defect in conversion of procollagen to collagen in a form of Ehlers–Danlos syndrome. *Science* **182**: 298.

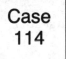

Charcot's Joint

Instruction

Examine this patient's joints.
Examine the locomotor system in this patient.

Salient features

- Enlargement of the affected joint (compare with the other side).
- Instability of the joint, in particular hypermobility of the joint.
- May be warm, swollen and tender in the early stages.

- Enlargement and crepitus may be present in the later stages.
- Check sensation in the affected limb.
- Tell the examiner that you would like to investigate as follows:
  Do a thorough neurological examination, looking for loss of proprioception and/or pain sensation.
  Examine the urine for sugar (looking for evidence of diabetes mellitus).
  Ask for lancinating pains, check posterior column signs and look for Argyll Robertson pupil (tabes dorsalis).
  Check for dissociated sensory loss (syringomyelia).

Questions

What do you understand by the term 'Charcot's joint'?

It is a chronic progressive degenerative arthropathy resulting from a disturbance in the sensory innervation of the affected joint. It is a neuropathic arthropathy which represents a complication of various disorders affecting the nervous system.

Mention a few conditions responsible for development of Charcot's joints.

- Diabetic neuropathy – affecting tarsal joints, tarsometatarsal, metatarsophalangeal joints.
- Tabes dorsalis – affecting knee, hip, ankle, lumbar and lower dorsal vertebrae.
- Syringomyelia – affecting shoulder, elbow, cervical vertebra.
- Myelomeningocoele – affecting ankle, tarsus.
- Miscellaneous: hereditary sensory neuropathies; peripheral nerve injury; congenital insensitivity to pain; leprosy.

Jean Martin Charcot (1825–1893) was a French neurologist. He was Professor of Pathology in 1872 and Professor of Nervous Diseases in 1882. The other conditions which bear his name include the following: Charcot's fever (intermittent fever due to cholangitis); Charcot's triad (intention tremor, nystagmus and scanning speech seen in multiple sclerosis); Charcot–Leyden crystals (seen in the sputum of asthmatics); Charcot–Marie–Tooth disease (peroneal muscular atrophy); Charcot–Wilbrand syndrome (visual agnosia).

References

Sinha, S, Munichoodappa, CS & Kozak, GP (1972) Neuroarthropathy (Charcot joints) in diabetes mellitus: clinical study in 101 cases. *Medicine* **51**: 191–210.

Case 115   Still's Disease

Instruction

Examine this patient's joints.
Look at this patient.

Salient features

- Micrognathia.
- Joints usually involved are upper cervical apophyseal joints, carpometacarpal joints and terminal interphalangeal joints.
- Maculopapular rash.
- Splenomegaly and lymph node enlargement.

- Tell the examiner that you would like to take a history of fever in the initial stages of the disease.

Questions

What do you know about juvenile chronic arthritis?

The diagnosis is made when a child less than 16 years of age has arthritis for at least 6 weeks with no other apparent cause. After 6 months of disease three major patterns are seen:

- Still's disease (10–20% of the cases) is defined as arthritis associated with daily temperature spikes to 39.4°C (103°F) for at least 2 weeks with or without maculopapular rash.
- Polyarticular juvenile chronic arthritis (15–25%) in which five or more joints are affected. Early fusion of the mandible and cervical spine result in a receding chin and early fusion of the cervical spine.
- Pauciarticular juvenile chronic arthritis (60–75%) which affects four or less joints; iritis is common in girls whereas sacroiliitis is common in boys.

What is the risk of treating young children with salicylates?

Reye's syndrome has been reported in children treated with aspirin for fever accompanying viral infections such as influenza. Children with juvenile chronic arthritis who are treated continuously for long periods of time have not been shown to have an increased incidence of this syndrome.

What are the poor prognostic factors?

- Chronic and polyarticular arthritis, particularly in patients with a systemic or pauciarticular onset.
- Polyarticular onset and a positive test for IgM rheumatoid factor.

Which drugs have been used in the treatment of resistant juvenile rheumatoid arthritis?

- Pencillamine.
- Hydroxychloroquine.
- Methotrexate (long-term therapy should be avoided as it is known to cause hepatic fibrosis).

Sir George Fredrick Still (1868–1941), a London physician, described 12 children (in 1897) who had a polyarthritis which he stated should be distinguished from rheumatoid arthritis, and another 6 children with a disease indistinguishable from adult rheumatoid arthritis. The distinctive findings in the first group included splenomegaly, lymphadenopathy, frequent occurrence of pericarditis and a predilection for cervical spine involvement. He also noted that fever and growth retardation were prominent features. The rash, however, was first described by Eric GL Bywaters.
RDK Reye (1912–1977), Australian histopathologist.

References

Starko, KM, Ray, CG, Dominquez, LB et al (1980) Reye's syndrome and salicylate use. *Pediatrics* **66:** 859.
Still, GF (1897) On a form of chronic joint disease in childhood. *Med Chir Trans* **80:** 47.
White, PH & Ansell, BM (1992) Methotrexate for juvenile rheumatoid arthritis. *N Engl J Med* **326:** 1077.

ENDOCRINOLOGY

Examination of the Thyroid

Instruction

Examine the thyroid.
Test this patient's thyroid status.
Look at the neck.

Salient features

- Introduce yourself to the patient and while shaking hands note whether his or her palms are warm and sweaty.
- *Inspection* of the neck:
    Look for the JVP.
    Scars of surgery.
    Enlarged cervical lymph nodes.
    Goitre.
- *Palpation* (always begin by palpating from behind):
    Seat the patient comfortably.
    Comment first on exophthalmos.
    While palpating the gland ensure that there is a glass of water to swallow.
    Palpate the thyroid and note the following:
        Size.
        Mobility
        Texture – simple or nodular (solitary or multiple)?
        Tenderness.
    Pemberton's sign (on raising the arms above the head patients with retrosternal goitres may develop signs of compression, i.e. suffusion of the face, syncope or giddiness).
    Palpate cervical lymph nodes.
    Feel the carotid arteries.
    Palpate for tracheal deviation.
    Percuss for retrosternal extension.

Auscultate over the gland for bruit, carotid bruits.
Test sternomastoid function (this muscle may be infiltrated in thyroid malignancies).

- Thyroid *function* should then be assessed:

1. Eye signs:
   Lid lag.
   Exophthalmos.
   Lid retraction (sclera visible above the cornea).
   Extraocular movements.
2. Hands:
   Pulse for tachycardia or atrial fibrillation.
   Tremor.
   Acropachy or clubbing.
   Palmar erythema (thyrotoxicosis).
   Supinator jerks (inverted in hypothyroidism).
   Proximal weakness in the upper arm.
3. Skin: look for pretibial myxoedema.
4. Elicit the ankle jerks.

If you are permitted to ask questions, inquire about shortness of breath and dysphagia.

Case 116   Graves' Disease

Instruction

Look at this patient.
Determine this patient's thyroid status.

Salient features

- Patient is fidgety and restless.
- While shaking hands with the patient note the warm sweaty palms.

- Look for tremor, thyroid acropachy, onycholysis (Plummer's nails) and palmar erythema.
- Check pulse (for tachycardia or the irregularly irregular pulse of atrial fibrillation).
- Comment on proptosis (after looking at the eyes from behind and above).
- Check for lid lag.
- Check for scars of previous tarsorrhaphy.
- Examine the neck for goitre and auscultate over the gland.
- Mention previous thyroidectomy scar if present.
- Comment on vitiligo if present.
- Check the shins for pretibial myxoedema (bilateral pinkish, brown dermal plaques).
- Test for proximal myopathy.
- Tell the examiner that you would like to ask the patient about the following:
    Easy irritability.
    Weight loss with increased appetite.
    Frequent defecation.
    Oligomenorrhoea.
    Dislike for hot weather.
    Family history of thyroid disease.

Questions

How would you confirm the diagnosis in this patient?

Thyroxine (T_4), thyroid-stimulating hormone (TSH) and thyroid autoantibodies.

What are the causes of hyperthyroidism?

- Primary: Graves' disease, toxic nodule, multinodular goitre, Hashimoto's thyroiditis, iodine-induced, excess thyroid hormone replacement, postpartum thyroiditis.
- Secondary: pituitary or excess TSH hypersecretion, hydatidiform moles, struma ovarii, factitious.

What are components of Graves' disease?

Hyperthyroidism with goitre, eye changes and pretibial myxoedema – they run independent courses.

What drugs are used in the treatment of thyrotoxicosis?

- Carbimazole.

- Methimazole.
- Propylthiouracil.

What are the disadvantages of antithyroid drugs?

- High rate of relapse once treatment is discontinued.
- Occasionally complicated by troublesome hypersensitivity reaction and very rarely by life-threatening agranulocytosis and hepatitis.

What are the advantages and disadvantages of radioactive iodine, when compared with partial thyroidectomy for thyrotoxicosis?

Both radioactive iodine therapy and surgical thyroidectomy are extremely effective and usually result in permanent cure. Patients will require lifelong thyroxine replacement. Thyroid surgery is expensive, inconvenient, occasionally complicated by injury to surrounding structures in the neck in less skilled hands, and complicated by the risks of anaesthesia.

Radioactive iodine, although safe, may not be acceptable to patients who are sensitive to the calamities of Chernobyl and Hiroshima.

Robert James Graves (1796–1853) was a Dublin physician who described this condition. HS Plummer (1874–1936), physician at the Mayo Clinic, Rochester, Minnesota; he also described Plummer–Vinson syndrome (iron deficiency anaemia and dysphagia).

References

Ladenson, PW (1991) Treatment for Graves' disease – letting the thyroid rest. *N Engl J Med* **324**: 989.

| Case 117 | Exophthalmos |

Instruction

Examine this patient's face.
Perform a general examination of this patient.

Salient features

- Prominent eyeballs.
- Look at the patient's eyes from behind and above for proptosis.
- Comment on lid retraction (the sclera above the upper limbus of the cornea will be seen); this is Dalrymple's sign.
- Comment on the sclera visible between the lower eyelid and the lower limbus of the cornea (i.e. comment on the exophthalmos). Most patients have bilateral exophthalmos with unilateral prominence.
- Check for lid lag (ask the patient to follow your finger and then move your finger along the arc of a circle from a point above his or her head to a point below the nose – the movement of the lid lags behind the globe); this is von Graefe's sign.
- Check for extraocular movements and comment on the cornea.
- Look for the following:
    Signs of thyrotoxicosis (fast pulse rate, tremor, sweating).
    Goitre (listen for bruit).
    Post-thyroidectomy scar.

Questions

What eye signs of thyroid disease do you know?

Werner's mnemonic, NO SPECS:
    No signs or symptoms.
    Only signs of upper lid retraction and stare with or without lid lag and exophthalmos.

    Soft tissue involvement.
    Proptosis.
    Extraocular muscle involvement.
    Corneal involvement.
    Sight loss due to optic nerve involvement.

How would you investigate this patient?

- History and clinical examination for signs of thyrotoxicosis and thyroid enlargement and bruit.
- Serum T_4, triiodothyronine (T_3), TSH.
- Thyroid antibodies.

What are the causes of unilateral exophthalmos?

Thyroid disease (seen in about 15% of cases), haemangiomas, lymphomas.

Mention the factors implicated in the phenomenon of lid lag.

* Sympathetic overstimulation, causing overaction of Müller's muscle.
* Myopathy of the inferior rectus causing overaction of superior rectus and levator muscles.
* Restrictive myopathy of the levator muscle.

What is euthyroid Graves' disease?

The patient will be clinically and biochemically euthyroid but will have manifestations of Graves' ophthalmopathy. A TRH stimulation test will show a flat response curve.

What would you recommend if a patient with unilateral exophthalmos is clinically and biochemically euthyroid?

* Ophthalmology referral.
* Ultrasound of the orbit.
* CT scan of the orbit.

How would you manage a patient with Graves' ophthalmopathy?

The single most important aspect is close liaison between the physician and the ophthalmologist.

Severe Graves' disease and visual loss should be immediately treated with high doses of corticosteroids, plasma exchange as an adjunct and if no improvement within 72–96 hours then orbital nerve decompression by surgical removal of the floor and medial wall of the orbit.

Moderate ophthalmopathy improves substantially in 2–3 years in most patients. In the interim the patient is treated symptomatically:

* Pain and grittiness is treated with methylcellulose eye drops by day and a lubricating eye ointment at night.
* Exposure keratitis may be relieved by lateral tarsorrhaphy, surgery of the lower eyelid.
* Diplopia may be relieved by prisms or surgery of the extraocular muscles.
* Static or worsening ophthalmopathy is an indication for steroids, orbital decompression or orbital irradiation.
* Patients should be advised to stop smoking.

Mild ophthalmopathy should be rectified by cosmetic eyelid surgery. It is important to remember that patients can be distressed by their appearance.

Does the treatment for hyperthyroidism affect Graves' ophthalmopathy?

Yes. Ophthalmopathy caused by Graves' disease may first appear or worsen during or after treatment for hyperthyroidism; iodine-131 is more likely to cause this as compared with antithyroid drugs or surgery.

J Dalrymple (1804–1852), English ophthalmologist.
Anthony Toft, endocrinologist, is the President of the Royal College of Physicians of Edinburgh.

References

DeJuan jun., E, Hurley, DP & Sapira, JD (1980) Racial differences in normal values of proptosis. *Arch Intern Med* **140**: 1230.
Fleck, BW & Toft, AD (1990) Graves' ophthalmopathy. *Br Med J* **300**: 1352.
Gorman, CA (1972) Unusual manifestation of Graves' disease. *Mayo Clin Proc* **47**: 926.
Hales, IB & Rundle, FF (1960) Ocular change in Graves' disease. A long term follow up study. *Q J Med* **29**: 113.
Hamburger, JI & Sugar, S (1972) What the internist should know about the ophthalmopathy of Graves' disease. *Arch Intern Med* **129**: 131.
Tallstedt, L, Lundell, G, Torring, O, Wallin, G et al (1992) Occurrence of ophthalmopathy after treatment for Graves' hyperthyroidism. *N Engl J Med* **326**: 1733.
Werner, SC (1977) Classification of the eye changes of Graves' disease. *J Clin Endocrinol Metab* **44**: 203.

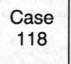

| Case 118 | Pretibial Myxoedema |

Instruction

Look at this patient's legs.

Salient features

- Red, thickened swellings above the lateral malleoli – peau d'orange appearance – which progresses to thickened, nonpitting oedema of the feet.

- Examine the following:
    The hands for acropachy, palmar erythema and warm, sweaty nature.
    The neck for goitre and thyroidectomy scar.
    The eyes for exophthalmos.
    The pulse for tachycardia and atrial fibrillation.
- Tell the examiner that you would like to know whether or not the patient has had any treatment, in particular radioactive iodine.

Questions

What investigations would you do?

Serum T_4, T_3 and TSH.

How are these lesions treated?

Intralesional steroids or fluorinated corticosteroids applied under polythene occlusion.

Mention a few symptoms which would indicate hyperthyroidism.

Excessive sweating, preference for cold weather, increased appetite and weight loss, nervousness, tiredness and palpitations, increased bowel movement.

How can hyperthyroidism present in the elderly?

Thyrotoxicosis can present in the elderly with atrial fibrillation, and such patients may lack other common signs of thyrotoxicosis; this is known as apathetic hyperthyroidism.

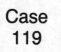

Case 119   Hypothyroidism

Instruction

Look at this patient's neck.
Look at this patient.
Do a general examination.

Salient features

- Coarse, dry skin (look for yellow skin of carotenaemia).
- Puffy lower eyelids.
- Loss of outer third of eyebrows, xanthelasma.
- Slow pulse.

- Examine the neck for goitre and the scar of previous thyroidectomy.
- Check the ankle jerks, looking for delayed relaxation.
- Tell the examiner that you would like to check for the following:
  Proximal muscle weakness.
  Cerebellar signs.
  Carpal tunnel syndrome.
- Tell the examiner that you would like to take a history of the following:
  Cold interolerance.
  Change in the voice (hoarse, husky).
  Lethargy, undue tiredness.
  Constipation.
  Moderate weight gain in spite of a loss of appetite.
  Menorrhagia.
  Radioiodine therapy for previous Graves' disease (the patient may have associated eye signs of Graves' disease).

Questions

How is delayed relaxation best elicited in the ankle?

Get the patient to kneel on a chair with his or her hands holding the back of the chair and then elicit the jerks on either side.

What are the causes of goitre?

- Idiopathic (majority).
- Hashimoto's thyroiditis.
- Graves' disease.
- Iodine deficiency (simple goitre).
- Puberty, pregnancy, subacute thyroiditis, goitrogens (lithium, phenylbutazone).

What is the thyroid status in Hashimoto's disease?

Hypothyroidism (usually).

What is the single best clinical indicator in hypothyroidism?

Delayed ankle jerks.

What is the best laboratory indicator for hypothyroidism?

Serum TSH levels.

How would you investigate a simple goitre?

Serum T_3, T_4, TSH and thyroid antibodies.

■ What is the cause for delayed relaxation in hypothyroidism?

The exact cause is not known. It is probably due to decreased muscle metabolism.

How would you investigate a nodular goitre?

- *Ultrasound* of the thyroid gland indicates whether goitre is *cystic* or *solid*.
- If *solid*, perform an *isotope scan* to indicate hot or cold nodule.
- If *hot nodule*, T_3, T_4, TSH.
- If *cold nodule*, fine needle aspiration.

How would you manage this patient with hypothyroidism?

Oral thyroxine replacement therapy for life. The therapeutic doses vary between 100 and 200 μg per day taken as a single dose. Dose adjustments are made once in every 3–4 weeks. The dose is adjusted depending on the clinical response and the suppression of elevated serum TSH levels.

What is the hazard in treating the elderly?

Rapid T_4 replacement may precipitate angina and myocardial infarction. The starting dose in the elderly is 50 μg per day.

What are the neurological manifestations of hypothyroidism?

- Carpal tunnel syndrome, peripheral neuropathy.
- Myxoedema madness.
- Myxoedema coma.
- Cerebellar syndrome.
- Pseudodementia.
- Hoffmann's syndrome, i.e. muscle aches with myotonia in myxoedema.

What other conditions are associated with Hashimoto's thyroiditis?

- Addison's disease.
- Diabetes mellitus.
- Graves' disease.
- Hypoparathyroidism.
- Premature ovarian failure.
- Pernicious anaemia.
- Rheumatoid arthritis.
- Sjögren's syndrome.
- Ulcerative colitis.
- SLE.
- Haemolytic anaemia.

H Hashimoto (1881–1934), Japanese surgeon.
Johann Hoffmann (1857–1919), German neurologist.

| Case 120 | Cushing's Syndrome |

Instruction

Examine this patient.
Look at this patient's face.

Salient features

- Moon-like facies, acne, hirsutism and plethora.
- Examine the following:
    The mouth for superimposed thrush.
    The interscapular area for 'buffalo hump'.
    The abdomen for purple striae (also seen over shoulders, thighs) and truncal obesity, scars of adrenalectomy.
    The limbs for wasting of the limbs, weakness of the muscles of the shoulders and hips – get the patient to squat (proximal myopathy) – and bruising.
- Tell the examiner that you would like to investigate as follows:
    Ask the patient if he or she has back pain and then examine the spine, looking for evidence of osteoporosis and collapse of vertebra, kyphoscoliosis.
    Test the urine for glucose.
    Measure the blood pressure.
    Ask the patient if he or she is on steroids.
    Check visual fields (for pituitary tumour).
    Fundus for optic atrophy, papilloedema, signs of hypertensive or diabetic retinopathy.

Note. Hirsutism is not common in Cushing's syndrome caused by exogenous steroids since they suppress adrenal androgen secretion.

Questions

Mention some causes of Cushing's syndrome.

- Steroids, including ACTH.
- Pituitary adenoma (Cushing's disease).
- Adrenal adenoma.
- Adrenal carcinoma.
- Ectopic ACTH by oat cell carcinoma of the lung.

Mention some conditions which are treated with long-term steroids?

- Rheumatoid arthritis.
- Asthma.
- SLE.
- Fibrosing alveolitis.

What is the difference between Cushing's disease and Cushing's syndrome?

Cushing's disease is increased production of steroids by the adrenals secondary to excess pituitary ACTH, whereas Cushing's syndrome is caused by excess steroid due to any cause.

■ How would you investigate such a patient?

Tests to *confirm the diagnosis*:

- 24-hour urinary free cortisol.
- Overnight dexamethasone test.
- Plasma cortisol at 9am and 10pm.

Tests to *determine the site of hormone overproduction*:

- Low- and high-dose dexamethasone test: low-dose dexamethasone test fails to suppress urinary steroid secretion in Cushing's disease, whereas high-dose dexamethasone (2 mg Q6H for 2 days) suppresses at least 50% of urinary steroid excretion.
- CXR for carcinoma of the bronchus.
- Plain X-ray of the abdomen for adrenal calcification.
- Ultrasound of the abdomen for adrenal tumours.
- If Cushing's disease is suspected:
  Plasma ACTH, X-ray of pituitary, MRI with gadolinium enhancement and bilateral measurements of corticotrophin in the inferior petrosal sinus.
  Corticotrophin-releasing hormone (CRH) test (helpful in distinguishing pituitary-led Cushing's disease from ectopic corticotrophin secretion).

What is pseudo Cushing's syndrome?

In chronic alcoholics and depression there may be increased urinary excretion of steroids, absent diurnal variation of plasma steroids and positive overnight dexamethasone test. All these investigations return to normal on discontinuation of alcohol or improvement of emotional status.

Harvey Williams Cushing (1869–1939) was a Professor of Surgery at Harvard. He was awarded the Pulitzer Prize for his biography of Osler.

References

Butler, PW & Besser, GM (1968) Pituitary-adrenal function in severe depressive illness. *Lancet* 1: 1234.

Cushing, H (1932) The basophil adenomas of the pituitary body and their clinical manifestation. *Bull Johns Hopkins Hosp* 1: 137.

Editorial (1990) CRH test in the 1990s. *Lancet* 336: 1416.

Klibanski, A & Zervas, NT (1991) Seminars in medicine of the Beth Israel Hospital, Boston: diagnosis and management of hormone-secreting pituitary adenomas. *N Engl J Med* 324: 822–830.

O'Riordan, JL, Blanshard, GP, Moxham, A et al (1966) Corticotrophin-secreting carcinomas. *Q J Med* 35: 137.

| Case 121 | Addison's Disease |

Instruction

Look at this patient who presented with weakness, loss of appetite and weight loss.

Salient features

- The striking abnormality is hyperpigmentation.
- Examine:
    The hand: compare the creases with your own.
    The mouth and lips for pigmentation.
    Areas not usually covered by clothing; nipples; areas irritated by belts, straps, collars or rings.
    Look for vitiligo.
- Tell the examiner that you would like to investigate as follows:
    Ask if the patient has been sitting in the sun.
    Examine the blood pressure, in particular for postural hypotension.
    Ask questions regarding fatigue, weakness, apathy, anorexia, nausea, vomiting, weight loss and abdominal pain.
    Examine the abdomen for adrenal scar (if the scar is pigmented, think of Nelson's syndrome and examine field defects).
- If you suspect Addison's disease tell the examiner that you would like to do a short tetracosactrin (synacthen) test.

Questions

Mention some causes of hyperpigmentation.

- Suntan.
- Race.
- Uraemia.
- Haemochromatosis.
- Primary biliary cirrhosis.
- Ectopic ACTH.
- Porphyria cutanea tarda.

- Nelson's syndrome.
- Malabsorption syndromes.

■ Mention some causes of Addison's disease.

- 80% idiopathic.
- Tuberculosis.
- Metastasis.
- HIV infection.

Which conditions may be associated with Addison's disease?

Graves' disease, Hashimoto's thyroiditis, primary ovarian failure, pernicious anaemia, hypoparathyroidism, polyglandular syndromes.

How would you investigate this patient?

- FBC (for lymphocytosis, eosiniphilia).
- Electrolytes (for hyponatraemia, hyperkalaemia, hyperchloraemic acidosis, hypercalcaemia).
- Blood glucose, looking for hypoglycaemia.
- Short tetracosactrin (synacthen) test; if positive, follow up with a prolonged ACTH stimulation test.
- ACTH and cortisol levels.
- Adrenal autoantibodies.
- CXR for TB.
- Plain X-ray of the abdomen for adrenal calcification.
- CT scan of adrenals.

How would you manage this patient if the underlying aetiology is autoimmune?

- Replacement steroids: prednisolone 5 mg mane and 2.5 mg nocte; adjust dose depending on serum levels and clinical wellbeing.
- Fludrocortisone 0.025–0.15 mg daily; adjust dose depending on postural hypotension.
- Give steroid card and Medic Alert bracelet.
- Stress the importance of regular therapy, and increase the dose in the event of stress such as dental extraction or urinary tract infection. It is also important to tell the patient that this therapy is lifelong and that he or she should keep an ampoule of hydrocortisone at home.
- Follow up every 6 months.

Note. In Addisonian crisis intravenous fluids and hydrocortisone should be administered.

Thomas Addison (1793–1860) qualified from Edinburgh and worked at Guy's Hospital, London. He wrote *The Constitutional and Local Effects of the Disease of the Suprarenal Capsules*. Armand Trosseau in Paris labelled the disease 'maladie d'Addison'. Addison also first described morphoea.

References

Addison, T (1855) Disease of the suprarenal capsules. *London Med Gaz* **43:** 517 (the original description of this disease).
Vita, JA, Silverberg, SJ, Goland, RS et al (1985) Clinical clues to the causes of Addison's disease. *Am J Med* **78:** 461.

Case 122   Acromegaly

Instruction

Examine this patient's face.
This patient complains of excessive sweating; examine him (or her).
Examine this patient's hands.

Salient features

Hands:

- On shaking hands there is excessive sweating.
- Large hands with broad palms, spatulate fingers; there is an increase in the 'volume' of the hands.
- Look for evidence of carpal tunnel syndrome (tap over the flexor retinaculum for Tinel's sign).

Face:

- Prominent supraorbital ridges.
- Large nose and lips.
- Protrusion of the lower jaw (prognathism); ask the patient to clench his or her teeth and note the malocclusion and splaying of the teeth.
- Ask the patient to show his or her tongue and look for macroglossia and for impressions by the teeth on the edges of the tongue.
- Test for bitemporal hemianopia and optic atrophy.

- Tell the examiner you would like to examine the following:
    Chest for cardiomegaly, gynaecomastia and galactorrhoea.
    Axillae for skin tags (molluscum fibrosum) acanthosis nigricans (back, velvety papillomas).
    Abdomen for hepatosplenomegaly.
    Neck for goitre.
    Joints for arthropathy, i.e. osteoarthroses, chondrocalcinosis.
    Spine for kyphosis.
    Blood pressure for hypertension (present in 15% of cases).
    Urine for sugar (impaired glucose tolerance).
    Old photographs of the patient to compare.

Questions

Would you like to ask the patient a few questions?

Ask about any increase in size of shoes, gloves and hat, and if the wedding ring is tight.

Mention some causes of macroglossia.

- Acromegaly.
- Amyloidosis.
- Hypothyroidism.
- Down's syndrome.

How can this condition present?

One third of patients notice a change in their features; one third are noticed to have a change in their features by their GPs and the remaining one third have symptoms such as excessive sweating and visual difficulties.

What are the indicators of disease activity?

- Symptoms such as headache, increase in size of ring, shoe or dentures.
- Excessive sweating.
- Skin tags.
- Glycosuria.
- Hypertension.
- Increased loss of visual fields.

■ How would you investigate this patient?

Biochemical tests:

- Nonsuppressibility of growth hormone (GH) levels to less than 2 ng ml^{-1} after oral administration of 100 g glucose.

- Plasma insulin-like growth factor levels.
- Also T$_4$, serum prolactin, testosterone; evaluate pituitary function – static and dynamic tests.

X-rays:

- Pituitary fossa.
- Sinuses.
- Chest.
- Hands and foot.
- CT head scan.
- MRI scan (if available, it is more reliable than CT).

Other investigations:

- Formal perimetry.
- Obtain old photos.
- New photos of face, torso, hands on chest.
- ECG.
- Triple stimulation test – if hypopituitarism is suspected.

What therapeutic options are available?

- Neurosurgical intervention – typically transsphenoidal – is the primary therapeutic choice for almost all patients.
- Radiation therapy is a primary treatment option for a few patients who have acromegaly but are not surgical candidates.
- Octreotide and bromocriptine are valuable as adjunctive therapy.

Mention four common causes of death in such patients.

- Cardiac failure.
- Tumour expansion (mass effect and haemorrhage).
- Effects of hypertension.
- Degenerative vascular disease.

How would you classify pituitary tumours?

- Traditional classification (based on haematoxylin–eosin (H&E) staining):
  Basophilic: corticotrophic adenomas.
  Acidophilic: densely granulated prolactinomas.
  Chromophobic: majority of the prolactinomas; sparsely granulated GH-secreting tumours; TSH-secreting, gonadotrophin-secreting and nonsecreting tumours.
- Hardy classification (based on size and invasiveness):
  Stage I: microadenomas (less than 1 cm) which may cause hormonal secretion but do not cause hypopituitarism or structural problems.

Stage II: macroadenomas (larger than 1 cm) with or without suprasellar extension.

Stage III: macroadenomas which invade the floor of the sella and may cause sellar enlargement or suprasellar extension.

Stage IV: invasive macroadenomas with diffuse destruction of the sella with or without suprasellar extension.

SR Bloom, contemporary Professor of Endocrinology, Hammersmith Hospital, whose chief interest is peptides.

References

Earll, JM, Sparks, LL & Forsham, PH (1967) Glucose suppression of serum growth hormone in the diagnosis of acromegaly. *JAMA* **201:** 628.

Klibanski, A & Zervas, NT (1991) Seminars in medicine of the Beth Israel Hospital, Boston: diagnosis and management of hormone-secreting pituitary adenomas. *N Engl J Med* **324:** 830.

McLachlan, MSF, Wright, AD & Doyle, FH (1970) Plain film and tomographic assessment of pituitary fossa in 140 acromegalic patients. *Br J Radiol* **43:** 360.

Melmed, S (1990) Acromegaly. *N Engl J Med* **322:** 967–975.

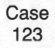

Case 123

Hypopituitarism (Simmonds' Disease)

Instruction

Look at this patient.

Salient features

- Patient is pale; the skin is soft.
- Paucity of axillary and pubic hair.

- Small testes in the male.
- Atrophy of breasts.

- Tell the examiner that you would like to investigate as follows:
    Examine the blood pressure for postural hypotension.
    Check visual fields; bitemporal hemianopia may be present.
    Examine the fundus for optic atrophy.
    Examine the external genitalia for hypogonadism.
    Take a history:
        In a male, of the frequency of shaving, impotence.
        In a female, of post partum haemorrhage, amenorrhoea.

Questions

Mention a few causes of hypopituitarism.

- Iatrogenic – from surgical removal of the pituitary or irradiation.
- Chromophobe adenoma (particularly in males).
- Postpartum pituitary necrosis (in females) – known as Sheehan's syndrome.

Rare cases:

- Craniopharyngioma.
- Metastatic tumours, granulomas (TB, sarcoid, haemochromatosis, histiocytosis X).

How would you assess such a patient?

- FBC for normochromic normocytic anaemia.
- U&E for hyponatraemia due to dilution.
- Measurement of pituitary hormone levels (ACTH, TSH, luteinising hormone (LH), GH, prolactin).
- Measurement of target organ secretion (T_4, T_3; serum cortisol, testosterone, oestrogen and progesterone levels).
- Pituitary stimulation tests:
    Thyrotrophin-releasing hormone (TRH) stimulation tests.
    Tetracosactrin (synacthen) tests.
    Insulin hypoglycaemia test.
    Luteinising hormone releasing hormone (LH–RH) tests.
- Skull X-ray.
- Assessment of visual fields (formal perimetry).

In what order do the hormone secretions generally fail?

In general GH, follicle-stimulating hormone (FSH) and LH secretions become deficient early, followed by TSH and ACTH. Last of all, ADH secretions diminish and fail.

Morris Simmonds of Hamburg described this condition in 1914.

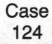

| Case 124 | Gynaecomastia |

Instruction

Look at this patient's chest.

Salient features

- Unilateral or bilateral enlargement of the breasts.
- Palpate to confirm presence of glandular tissue.
- Tell the examiner that you would like to investigate as follows:
    Look for stigmata of cirrhosis of the liver.
    Take a drug history – oestrogens, digoxin, spironolactone cimetidine, diazepam, alkylating agents, methyldopa, clomiphene.

Questions

Mention the physiological causes of gynaecomastia.

- Newborn.
- Adolescence.
- Ageing.

Mention a few pathological causes.

- Liver disease.
- Drugs.
- Thyrotoxicosis.
- Klinefelter syndrome.
- Viral orchitis.
- Renal failure.

■ What are the causes of a feminising state?

- Absolute increase in oestrogen formation by tumours.
- Increased availability of oestrogen precursors, e.g. as a result of cirrhosis.
- Increased extraglandular oestrogen synthesis.
- Relative increase in ratio of oestrogen to androgen, e.g. as a result of testicular failure.
- Drugs.

HF Klinefelter (b. 1912), American physician who worked at Johns Hopkins Hospital. He described this syndrome with Albright while he was a visiting Fellow at Harvard.

References

Wilson, JD (1991) Gynaecomastia. *N Engl J Med* **324**: 335.

| Case 125 | Carpopedal Spasm (Post-Thyroidectomy Hypoparathyroidism) |

Instruction

Look at this patient's hands.

Salient features

- Spasm of the hands – fingers are extended, except at the metacarpophalangeal joints, and the thumb is strongly adducted.

- Look at the feet for spasm and then investigate as follows:
  Tap over the facial nerve (in front of tragus of the ear) – there is contraction of the lips and facial muscles (Chvostek's sign).
  Look into the mouth for candidiasis (may be seen in primary hypoparathyroidism).
  Check for thyroidectomy scar.
  Look for cataracts.

- Tell the examiner that you would like to perform the following tests:
  Do a skull X-ray (looking for basal ganglia calcification).
  Check serum calcium and magnesium levels.

Questions

What is Trousseau's sign?

The cuff is inflated just above the systolic pressure for 3 minutes and this will cause the hand to go into spasm.

What are the causes of hypoparathyroidism?

- Damage during thyroid or neck surgery.
- Idiopathic.
- Destruction of the parathyroid gland due to the following:
  Radioactive iodine therapy.
  External neck irradiation.
  Haemochromatosis.
  Metastatic disease from breast, lung, lymphoproliferative disorder.

■ What do you know about pseudohypoparathyroidism?

It is a condition which is characterised by end-organ resistance to parathyroid hormone. The biochemistry is similar to idiopathic hypoparathyroidism except that patients with pseudohypoparathyroidism do not respond to injected parathyroid hormone. These patients are moon faced, short statured and mentally retarded and may have short fourth or fifth metacarpals.

Frantisek Chvostek (1835–1884) was a Professor of Medicine in Vienna, Austria.
Armand Trousseau (1801–1867) was a Parisian physician who was the first to refer to adrenal insufficiency as Addison's disease.

References

Davis, RH, Fourman, P & Smith, JWG (1960) Problems of parathyroid insufficiency after thyroidectomy. *Lancet* **2:** 1432.

Juan, D (1979) Hypocalcemia: differential diagnosis and mechanisms. *Arch Intern Med* **139:** 1166.

DERMATOLOGY

<table>
<tr><td>Case
126</td><td>Maculopapular Rash</td></tr>
</table>

Instruction

Would you like to perform a general examination of this patient.
Look at this patient.

Salient features

- Reddish, blotchy maculopapular rash over the trunk (check the chest, back and axillae) and limbs.

- Palpate the surface of the rash to confirm your inspectory findings.
- Check the mucous membranes of the mouth.
- Tell the examiner that you would like to ask the patient some questions:
    Ask whether or not the rash itches.
    Ask where the rash started and ask the patient to describe its evolution.
    Take a drug history.
    Examine for lymph nodes (glandular fever) – some examiners may expect you to examine lymph nodes as a part of general

examination. If lymph nodes are palpable then examine all groups (cervical, supraclavicular, axillary and inguinal).

Note. Avoid waffling descriptions such as 'skin rash'.

Questions

What is your differential diagnosis?

- Drug-induced rash (e.g. ampicillin, cephalosporins).
- Glandular fever.

What is your differential diagnosis when the rash is associated with lymphadenopathy?

- Glandular fever.
- Lymphoproliferative disorders such as Hodgkin's disease.
- HIV infection.

Case 127	Purpura

Instruction

Examine this patient's skin.

Salient features

- There may be small circumscribed bleeding into the skin – purpura or larger lesions – bruises or ecchymoses.
- Look for an underlying cause.
- Comment on the patient's age – consider senile purpura.
- Comment on the distribution – Henoch–Schoenlein purpura is seen over the buttocks and lower limbs (page 267).

- Look for the following signs:
  Rheumatoid arthritis where purpura is drug-induced (steroids, gold).
  Anaemia – (leukaemia, marrow aplasia or infiltration).
  Chronic liver disease.
  Ulcers in the mouth (severe neutropenia).
  Bleeding gums, corkscrew hair of scurvy (particularly in the elderly).
  Stigmata of Ehlers–Danlos syndrome.
  Bleeding from multiple venepuncture sites (disseminated intravascular coagulation).
- Tell the examiner that you would like to investigate as follows:
  Take a drug history – steroids, anticoagulants, carbimazole, phenylbutazone, chloramphenicol.
  Examine for spleen, liver and lymph nodes.

Questions

What are the common causes of purpura?

- Senile purpura, due to senile changes in the vessel walls.
- Purpura induced by steroids or anticoagulants.
- Thrombocytopenia due to leukaemia and marrow aplasia.

What do you know about Moschowitz's syndrome?

Moschowitz syndrome or thrombotic thrombocytopenic purpura is an acute disorder characterised by thrombocytopenic purpura, microangiopathic haemolytic anaemia, transient and fluctuating neurological features, fever and renal impairment.

What are the causes of bruising?

- Thrombocytopenia: idiopathic thrombocytopenic purpura, marrow replacement by leukaemia or secondary infiltration.
- Vascular defects: senile purpura, steroid-induced purpura, Henoch–Schoenlein purpura, scurvy, von Willebrand's disease, uraemia.
- Coagulation defects: haemophilia, anticoagulants, Christmas disease.
- Drugs: thiazides, sulphonamides, phenylbutazone, sulphonylureas, sulindac, barbiturates.

E Moschowitz (1879–1964), New York physician.
EH Henoch (1820–1910), German paediatrician.
JL Schoenlein (1793–1864) was successively Professor of Medicine in Würzburg, Zurich and Berlin.

Case 128	Psoriasis

Instruction

Look at this patient.
Do a general examination.

Salient features

- Well-demarcated salmon pink plaques with silvery white scales over extensor surfaces, scalp, navel and natal cleft.
- Look at the nails for pitting.
- Tell the examiner that you would like to take a history of joint pains.

Questions

How common is this condition?

It affects 1–2% of the population of the UK.

What are the types of psoriasis?

- Chronic plaque psoriasis.
- Guttate psoriasis.
- Pustular psoriasis – localised or generalised.
- Erythrodermic psoriasis.

Mention a few drugs which may aggravate or precipitate psoriasis.

Alcohol, beta blockers, NSAIDs, lithium, chloroquine, mepacrine.

How would you assess the severity of psoriasis?

- The patient's own perception of the disability.
- Objective assessment of disability.

What treatment modalities are available?

- Topical: coal tar, dithranol, steroids.
- Phototherapy with ultraviolet B (PUVA B).

- Systemic treatment: photochemotherapy (PUVA), methotrexate, retinoids, cyclosporin, hydroxyurea, azathioprine, systemic steroids.

What are the indications for systemic treatment?

- Failure of topical therapy.
- Repeated hospital admissions for topical treatment.
- Extensive plaque psoriasis in the elderly.
- Generalised pustular or erythrodermic psoriasis.
- Severe psoriatic arthropathy.

References

Williams, REA (1991) Guidelines for management of patients with psoriasis. *Br Med J* **303:** 829.

Case 129	Bullous Eruption

Instruction

Look at this patient.

Salient features

- Bullous eruption.

- Comment on the distribution: knee, thighs, forearms and umbilicus in the elderly (pemphigoid).

- Look in the mouth for ulceration; if blisters break easily, leaving denuded skin, it is more likely to be pemphigus.

- Tell the examiner that a biopsy of the skin is essential to confirm the diagnosis.

Questions

What do you understand by the term 'bulla'?

It is a circumscribed elevation of the skin, larger than 0.5 cm and containing fluid.

How would you confirm the diagnosis?

A biopsy of a fresh blister (less than 12 hours old) with a portion of perilesional skin for histology and immunofluorescent studies.

Mention a few blistering conditions.

● Common: friction, insect bites, drugs, burns, impetigo, contact dermatitis.
● Uncommon: pemphigoid, pemphigus vulgaris, dermatitis herpetiformis, bullous erythema multiforme, epidermolysis bullosa, porphyria cutanea tarda.

How would you manage a patient with pemphigus vulgaris?

Barrier nursing, antibiotics, intravenous fluids, large doses of systemic steroids, usually with immunosuppressive drugs – azathioprine, cyclophosphamide or methotrexate – which act as steroid sparing agents.

What are the characteristics of pemphigus vulgaris?

Pemphigus vulgaris is characterised by bullae in the epidermis. It is often preceded by bullae in the mucous membrane. Superficial separation of the skin after pressure, trauma or on rubbing the thumb laterally on the surface of uninvolved skin may cause easy separation of the epidermis (Nikolsky's sign). Biopsy shows disruption of epidermal intercellular connections called acantholysis. Immunofluorescence shows intercellular deposition of IgG in the epidermis.

What are the characteristics of bullous pemphigoid?

It is a relatively benign condition with remissions and exacerbations. The bullae are subepidermal and immunoelectron microscopy shows that deposits of IgG and complement 3 (C3) are found in the lamina lucida of the basement membrane.

PV Nikolsky (b.1858) Professor of Dermatology, first in Warsaw and later in Rostov.

| Case 130 | Henoch–Schoenlein Purpura |

Instruction

Look at this patient's legs.

Salient features

- Purpuric rash over the legs and buttocks.
- Tell the examiner that you would like to examine the rest of the body – including arms, body, scalp and behind the ears – for distribution of the rash.
- Examine the mouth in order to confirm or rule out involvement of mucous membranes.
- Tell the examiner that you would like to investigate as follows:
    Ask the patient about the following:
    Joint pains (knee and ankles are commonly involved).
    Abdominal pain.
    The rash – its onset and evolution.
    Recent drug ingestion.
    Examine the urine for haematuria.

Questions

What do you know about Henoch–Schoenlein purpura?

Henoch–Schoenlein or anaphylactoid purpura is a distinct, self-limiting vasculitis which occurs in children and young adults. It is a disorder characterised by nonthrombocytopenic purpura, arthralgia, abdominal pain and glomerular nephritis. It is due to circulating IgA-containing immune complexes. It usually lasts between 1 and 6 weeks and subsides without sequelae if the renal involvement is mild.

What investigations would you like to do?

- Examine the urine for haematuria and proteinuria.
- Antinuclear factor.
- VDRL.
- Skin biopsy to detect arteriolar and capillary vasculitis.

What is the differential diagnosis?

- Drug-induced purpura.
- SLE.
- Gonococcal arthralgia.
- Keratoderma blenorrhagicum.
- Secondary syphilis.

Eduard Heinric Henoch (1820–1910) qualified in Berlin, where he ran the neurology department: he studied under Schoenlein and eventually became a paediatrician. Johannes Lucas Schoenlein (1793–1864) qualified and became Professor of Medicine in Würzburg but because of his liberal views he was dismissed; he eventually became Professor of Medicine first in Zurich and then in Berlin.

References

Roth, DA, Wilz, DR & Theil, GB (1985) Schoenlein–Henoch syndrome in adults. *Q J Med* **55**: 145.

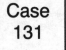

Ichthyosis

Instruction

Look at this patient.
Examine this patient's skin.
Perform a general examination of this patient.

Salient features

- Rough, dry skin with fish-like scales.
- Examine the palms for dry skin and hyperkeratotic creases.

- Tell the examiner that you would like to investigate as follows:
  Take a family history of the disorder.
  Ask whether or not this is of recent onset (underlying malignancy).

Questions

What do you know about ichthyosis?

Ichthyosis can be classified as follows:

1. *Inherited* ichthyosis is present from birth or childhood and may be apparent only in winter.
   - Ichthyosis vulgaris: present from childhood; autosomal dominant; spares flexural areas; associated atopy.
   - X-linked ichthyosis: present from birth; over the trunk; associated corneal opacities.
   - Lamellar ichthyosis: autosomal recessive; present from birth; seen over the body, palms and soles; associated ectropion.
   - Epidermolytic hyperkeratosis: autosomal dominant; present since birth; predominant flexural involvement.
2. *Metabolic* ichthyosis:
   - Refsum's disease – a metabolic disorder of lipid metabolism.
3. *Malignancy* – as a cutaneous marker:
   - Hodgkin's disease.
   - Multiple myeloma.
   - Cancer of the breast.

How would you manage such patients?

Regular use of emollients and moisturising creams. Creams containing urea are useful.

S Refsum, Norwegian physician.

Case	Hereditary Haemorrhagic
132	Telangiectasia (Rendu–Osler–
	Weber Disease)

Instruction

Examine this patient's face.
Do a general examination.
Look at this patient's face.

Salient features

- Punctiform lesions and dilated small vessels present on the face, in particular around the mouth.
- The patient may be pale.

- Look into the patient's mouth, and inspect the tongue and palate for telangiectasia.
- Tell the examiner that you would like to ask the patient two questions:
    Does it run in the family (autosomal dominant)?
    Is there a history of gastrointestinal bleeding?
- Tell the examiner that you would like to examine the chest for bruits (pulmonary arteriovenous malformations).

Questions

What do you understand by the term 'telangiectasia'?

Telangiectasia is a cluster of dilated capillaries and venules.

Mention a few conditions in which telangiectasia is seen.

- Of the face:
    Those who work outdoors in a temperate or cold climate (e.g. farmers).
    In mitral stenosis.
    Myxoedema.
    Transitory phenomenon during pregnancy.

- Other sites:
    Secondary to irradiation.
    Scleroderma (CREST syndrome).
    Dermatomyositis.
    SLE.
    Acne rosacea.
    Lupus pernio.
    Polycythaemia.
    Necrobiosis lipoidica diabeticorum.

What are the complications of hereditary telangiectasia?

- Epistaxis.
- Upper gastrointestinal haemorrhage.
- Haemoptysis due to pulmonary arteriovenous malformations.
- Iron deficiency anaemia.

How would you manage such patients?

- Ferrous sulphate for anaemia.
- Oestrogens have been reported to be helpful in epistaxis.

This condition was described by HJLM Rendu, a French physician, in 1896, Sir William Osler in 1901 and F Parkes Weber, London physician, in 1936.

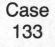

| Case 133 | Herpes Labialis |

Instruction

Look at this patient's mouth.

Salient features

- Small vesicles on the lips and around the mouth.
- Look for vesicles in the mouth.

Questions

What usually causes 'cold sore'?

Herpes simplex virus (HSV) type I: in children it causes asymptomatic gingivostomatitis; in adults there may be severe stomatitis with mouth ulcers, local lymph node enlargement and systemic features.

What do you know about HSV-II?

HSV-II causes genital infection, called vulvovaginitis. Women with genital herpes ought to have cervical screening as a link is suspected with carcinoma of the cervix.

What are complications of herpes infections?

- Erythema multiforme.
- Disseminated infection in the immunocompromised individual.
- Herpes keratitis, scarring and visual impairment.
- Herpes simplex encephalitis.
- Herpetic whitlow.
- Herpes simplex meningitis.

How would you treat herpes labialis?

Acyclovir cream applied locally.

Case 134	Herpes Zoster Syndrome (Shingles)

Instruction

Look at this patient.

Salient features

- Vesicular rash along a dermatome.
- Enlargement of the draining lymph gland.
- Tell the examiner that you would like to ask about the following:
  Pain particularly in the ophthalmic branch of the trigeminal, and in the lower thoracic dermatomes.
  Past history of shingles or chickenpox.
- Remember that the virus affects both the posterior horn of the spinal cord and the skin supplied by sensory fibres which pass through the diseased root ganglion.

Questions

In which layer of the skin are the vesicles formed?

They are formed in the prickle-cell layer of the epidermis as a result of the 'balloon degeneration' of the cells and serous exudation from the corium.

How does this condition present?

Pain in the distribution of the dermatome; malaise; fever, followed a few days later by a rash in the same distribution as the pain. Starts as macules then forms vesicles and then pustules.

How would you confirm the diagnosis?

The diagnosis is usually clinical. It is confirmed by rising viral titres and isolation of the virus is from the blister.

How would you manage such a patient?

- Topical idoxuridine 5% solution if caught in the first 36 hours of the eruption.
- Pain relief including amitriptyline in severe cases.
- Intravenous acyclovir in the immunocompromised individual.
- Interferon appears to be effective in limiting zoster in patients with cancer.

What are the complications of herpes zoster?

- Corneal ulcerations.
- Gangrene of the affected area.
- Phrenic nerve palsy.
- Meningoencephalitis.
- Ramsay Hunt syndrome.

- Postherpetic neuralgia.
- Disseminated zoster including pneumonia.

J Ramsay Hunt (1874–1937), US neurologist.

References

Esmann, V, Geil, JP, Kroon, S et al (1987) Prednisolone does not prevent post-herpetic neuralgia. *Lancet* 2: 126.

Case 135	Lichen Planus

Instruction

Look at this patient's skin.

Salient features

- Papular, purplish, flat-topped eruption with fine white streaks (Wickham's striae) over the anterior wrists and forearms, sacral region, legs and penis.
- Look into the mouth for lace-like pattern of white lines and papules. (Remember that oral lichen planus must be differentiated from leucoplakia.)
- Examine the scalp for cicatricial alopecia.
- Comment on the eruptions along linear scratch marks (Koebner's phenomenon).

Note. The three cardinal findings of lichen planus are the typical skin lesions, histopathological features of T cell infiltration of the dermis in a band pattern, and IgG and C3 fluorescence at the basement membrane at the dermis.

Questions

Mention a few conditions which present as white lesions in the mouth.

- Leucoplakia.
- Candidiasis.
- Aphthous stomatitis.
- Squamous papilloma.
- Verruca vulgaris.
- Secondary syphilis.

Mention a few conditions in which ulcers can be found in the mouth.

- Erosive lichen planus.
- Pemphigus vulgaris.
- Recurrent aphthous ulcers.
- Behçet's disease.
- Stevens–Johnson syndrome.
- Recurrent herpes simplex.

Do you know of any drugs which cause lichen planus?

- Gold, organic mercurials.
- Chloroquine, mepacrine.
- Methyldopa.
- Quinine.
- Chlorpropamide, tolbutamide.
- Topical contact with film developer.

What is the prognosis in lichen planus?

Lichen planus is a benign condition which lasts for months to years. It may be recurrent. Oral lesions may be persistent.

How would you manage these lesions?

- Local measures: local steroid creams or intralesional steroids.
- General measures: PUVA, isotretinoin, dapsone.

LS Wickham (1860–1913), French dermatologist.
H Koebner (1838–1904), German dermatologist.

References

Eisen, D, Ellis, CN, Duell, EA, Griffiths, CEM & Voorhees, JJ (1990) Effect of topical cyclosporin rinse on oral lichen planus. *N Engl J Med* **323**: 290–294.
Savin, JA (1991) Oral lichen planus. *Br Med J* **302**: 544–545.

Case 136	Vitiligo

Instruction

Look at this patient.

Salient features

- Hypopigmented patches which are distributed symmetrically; sometimes the border may be hyperpigmented.
- Look at the scalp for alopecia.
- Tell the examiner that you would like to ask whether or not it runs in the family.

Note. Scratching when the disease is active may induce lesions along the scratch marks; this is termed isomorphic response or Koebner's phenomenon.

Questions

Mention some associated conditions.

Organ-specific autoimmune conditions:

- Thyroid disease – Graves' disease, myxoedema, Hashimoto's disease.
- Pernicious anaemia.
- Diabetes mellitus.
- Alopecia areata.
- Addison's disease.

Which fungal condition can be mistaken for vitiligo?

Pityriasis versicolor (caused by the fungus *Malassezia furfur*).

How would you manage such patients?

- New lesions of vitiligo may benefit from topical steroids.
- PUVA therapy may be of benefit to some patients.

Note. On the whole, treatment of vitiligo remains unsatisfactory.

Mention a few conditions in which hypopigmentation is common.

- Hypopituitarism.
- Albinism.
- Phenylketonuria.
- Leprosy.
- Burns.
- Radiodermatitis.

H Koebner (1838–1904), German dermatologist.

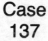

| Case 137 | Raynaud's Phenomenon |

Instruction

Examine this patient's hands.

Salient features

- Hands may be painful – ask the patient.
- The hands are cyanosed and cold or may be warm and red or blue.

- Examine the hands carefully for signs of scleroderma (tightening of skin, telangiectasia).
- Examine the face for tightening of skin around the mouth (scleroderma), butterfly rash (SLE).
- Tell the examiner you would like to ask the patient about the following:
    The different phases of Raynaud's phenomenon (in idiopathic Raynaud's the cold, dead-white hands become blue and finally red and painful).
    Occupation (polishing tools, vibrating tools).
    Dysphagia (CREST syndrome).

Butterfly rash, arthralgia, xerostomia (SLE, collagen vascular disorder).
Use of electrically heated gloves.
- Tell the examiner you would like to examine upper limb pulses and blood pressure in both upper limbs (useful in the detection of cervical rib).

Questions

What are the causes of Raynaud's phenomenon?

- Immunological and connective tissue disorders:
  Scleroderma.
  SLE.
  Dermatomyositis.
  Rheumatoid arthritis.
  Mixed connective tissue disorders.
- Obliterative arterial disease:
  Atherosclerosis.
  Thoracic outlet syndrome, cervical rib.
- Occupational:
  Vibration, causing white fingers.
  Cold injury, e.g. from handling frozen commodities.
  Vinyl chloride.
- Drugs:
  Beta blockers.
  Bromocriptine.
  Sulphasalazine.
  Ergot alkaloids.
- Miscellaneous:
  Cold agglutinins.
  Cryoglobulins.
  Idiopathic.

■ Do you know the factors involved in Raynaud's phenomenon?

Calcitonin-gene-related peptide (CGRP) is deficient.

What drugs have been used to treat Raynaud's phenomenon?

Nifedipine, stanazol, inositol nicotinate, naftidrofuryl oxalate, prostaglandin I2, thymoxamine, guanethidine, prazosin.

Do you know any other vasospatic conditions?

- White finger syndrome.
- Livedo reticularis.

- Erythromelalgia.
- Chilblains.

Maurice Raynaud (1834–1881) described the sign in 1862. He was a physician at Hôpital Lariboisière, Paris.

References

Bunker, CB, Terenghi, G, Springall, DR, Polak, JM & Doud, PM (1990) Deficiency of CGRP in Raynaud's phenomenon. *Lancet* **336:** 1531.
Grigg, MH & Wolfe, JHN (1991) ABC of vascular diseases: Raynaud's syndrome and similar conditions. *Br Med J* **303:** 913.
Raynaud, M (1888) On local and symmetrical gangrene of the extremities. In Barlow T (translator) *Selected Monographs*, vol 121. London: New Sydenhan Society.

Case 138	Systemic Lupus Erythematosus

Instruction

Examine this patient's face (usually young female).

Salient features

- Butterfly rash – follicular plugging, scales, telangiectasia and scarring (the patient may be Cushingoid due to steriods).
- Examine the following areas:
  Conjunctiva for anaemia (often Coombs positive).
  Mouth for ulcers (seen in one third of cases).
  Scalp for alopecia.
  Sun-exposed areas and elbows for vasculitic rash, subcutaneous nodules.

Nails for splinter haemorrhages, nail fold capillaries and periungual infarcts.

Hands for palmar erythema, Raynaud's phenomenon, arthritis.

Knees for vasculitic rash.

Feet for oedema (secondary to nephrotic syndrome).

- Tell the examiner that you would like to examine the urine for proteinuria.

Questions

What are the skin manifestations of SLE?

Butterfly rash, periungual erythema, nail fold telangiectasia, alopecia, livedo reticularis, hyperpigmentation, urticaria, purpura, scarring eruption of discoid lupus.

What are the criteria for diagnosis of SLE?

Any four of the following eleven criteria are required to make a diagnosis:

- Malar rash.
- Discoid rash.
- Photosensitivity.
- Oral ulcers.
- Arthritis – nonerosive arthritis.
- Serositis – pleuritis, pericarditis.
- Renal involvement – proteinuria, cellular casts.
- Neurological involvement – seizures, psychosis.
- Haematological involvement – haemolytic anaemia, leucopenia, thrombocytopenia.
- Antinuclear antibody – seen in over 95% of patients.
- Immunological disorder – positive LE cell, anti-DNA antibody, false-positive syphilitic serology.

How would you manage a patient with SLE?

- Avoidance of sunlight provocation.
- Avoidance of drug provocation – penicillin, sulphonamides.
- Encourage the patient to join the Lupus Society.
- Medical treatment is largely empirical, selected on the basis of specific manifestations.
- No therapy is curative.

1. Serological abnormalities and minor cytopenias unaccompanied by symptoms need no treatment.
2. Rash and mild systemic symptoms are treated with antimalarial drugs.

3. Mild or moderate arthritis, fever or pleuropericarditis are treated with NSAIDs or low-dose prednisolone.
4. Malaise, weight loss and lymphadenopathy are treated with low-dose prednisone.
5. High fever, active inflammatory glomerulonephritis, severe thrombocytopenia, severe haemolytic anaemia and most neurological disturbances require treatment with high-dose prednisone (more than 60 mg per day for 4–6 weeks).
6. Rapidly progressive renal disease is treated by intravenous administration of a bolus of 1000 mg methylprednisolone.
7. Lupus glomerulonephritis with high histological activity score requires oral or intravenous cyclophosphamide with high-dose steroids.
8. Thromboembolism in patients with antiphospholipid antibody requires long-term anticoagulation.
9. Experimental treatments for severe disease include apharesis, intravenous γ-globulin, cyclosporin immunoadsorption, photochemotherapy, nodal irradiation and various monoclonal antibodies.

RRA Coombs (b.1921), Professor of Immunology at Cambridge, is reported to have said 'red blood cells were primarily designed by God as tools for the immunologist and only secondarily as carriers of haemoglobin'.

References

Harvey, AM, Shulman, LE, Tumulty, PA et al (1954) SLE: review of literature and clinical analysis of 138 cases. *Medicine* **33**: 291 (classic clinical description).
Lockshin, MD (1991) Therapy for SLE. *N Engl J Med* **324**: 180.
Tan, EM, Cohen, AS, Fries, JF et al (1982) The 1982 revised criteria for classification of SLE. *Arthritis Rheum* **25**: 1271.

Case 139	Phlebitis Migrans

Instruction

Look at this patient's leg; he (or she) has had similar lesions at different sites at intervals.

Salient features

- Inflamed superficial leg veins.

- Tell the examiner that you would like to investigate for underlying malignancy, usually carcinoma of the pancreas or stomach (Trousseau's sign).

Questions

In which other condition is superficial phlebitis a prominent sign?

Thromboangiitis obliterans.

What other dermatoses complicate pancreatic disease?

- Panniculitis.
- 'Bronze' pigmentation of haemochromatosis.
- 'Necrolytic migratory erythema' of glucagonoma syndrome.
- Cutaneous haemorrhage of acute pancreatitis – 'bruising' of the left flank (Grey Turner's sign) or umbilicus (Cullen's sign).

Armand Trousseau (1801–1867), physician, Hôtel-Dieu, Paris, noted the sign as his death warrant, confirming his suspicion of an underlying malignancy.

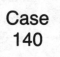

Case 140 — Erythema Multiforme

Instruction

Do a general examination.

Salient features

- Target-shaped skin lesions, usually over the limbs; pleomorphic eruption with macules, papules and bullae.
- Look at the mucous membranes of mouth and eyes (Stevens–Johnson syndrome).
- Tell the examiner that you would like to proceed as follows:
    Examine the external genitalia for ulcers.
    Take a history of preceding sore throat or cold.
    Take a drug history (barbiturates, sulphonamides).

Questions

What is the underlying aetiology?

- Herpes simplex infection.
- Mycoplasma infection.
- Streptococcal infection.
- Drug hypersensitivity.
- Collagen vascular disorder, e.g. SLE.
- Multiple myeloma.
- Idiopathic – in 50% of cases no cause may be found.

How would you investigate this patient?

- Viral titres, in particular for herpes simplex type I.
- Complement fixation test for mycoplasma.
- Antistreptolysin O (ASO) titres.

If the above are negative:

- Serum (s) autoantibodies.
- Protein electrophoresis, urine for Bence-Jones proteins.

What do you understand by the term 'Stevens–Johnson syndrome'?

Stevens–Johnson syndrome is a severe form of erythema multiforme with widespread bullous eruptions associated with oral and genital ulcerations and marked constitutional symptoms.

How would you manage patients with Stevens–Johnson syndrome?

Symptomatic treatment with antipyretics, intravenous fluids and antibiotics. The role of steroids is controversial. Erythema multiforme is a self-limiting condition, although Stevens–Johnson may be fatal.

FC Johnson (1894–1934) and AM Stevens (1884–1945), both American paediatricians, described this condition in 1922 in a paper titled 'A new eruptive fever with tonsillitis and ophthalmia'.
H Bence-Jones (1814–1873), English physician, St George's Hospital, London.

Case 141	Erythema Ab Igne

Instruction

Examine this patient's legs.
Examine this patient's abdomen.

Salient features

- Reticular erythematous or pigmented rash, usually on the forelegs (or abdomen), known as 'Granny's tartan'.
- Look for features of hypothyroidism (pulse, ankle jerks).
- Tell the examiner that you would like to proceed as follows:
  Ask the patient whether she exposed the affected area to heat.
  Measure T_4 and TSH levels.

Note. If the rash is present over the anterior abdominal wall or over the lumber region then it is very likely that there is an intra-abdominal malignancy.

Questions

How may erythema ab igne be complicated?

Epitheliomas may develop in keratoses which form in later stages of this condition.

What other reticulated rashes do you know?

- Livedo reticularis, seen in the following conditions:
  Polyarteritis nodosa.
  SLE.
  Occult malignant neoplasm.
  Atherosclerotic microemboli to the skin.
  Physiological in young women (it is best observed on the thighs of British school girls playing hockey in shorts on winter afternoons!).
- Cutaneous marmorta seen in children.

Mention some skin abnormalities related to heat or cold.

- Erythema ab igne.
- Livedo reticularis (due to cold in young women).
- Raynaud's phenomenon.
- Chilblains.

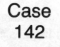

Case 142   Hirsutism

Instruction

Examine this patient.

Salient features

- Excessive hair growth particularly over the face and upper and lower limbs.
- Tell the examiner that you would like to proceed as follows:
  Take a menstrual history.
  Check the blood pressure, and the urine for sugar.
  Comment on Cushingoid features, if any.
  Look for signs of virilisation (receding hairline, breast atrophy, clitoromegaly).

Questions

Why do you want to take a menstrual history?

If the menstruation is normal it indicates that there is no increase in testosterone production. However, if menstruation is abnormal then the commonest cause is polycystic ovary disease (POCD) which is the underlying cause in 92% of the women with hirsutism (the popular belief that most cases of hirsutism are idiopathic is untrue).

What other causes of hirsutism can you tell us?

- Cushing's syndrome.
- Adrenal or ovarian tumours.
- Acromegaly.
- Drugs – phenytoin, minoxidil, androgens.

What is the relationship between body weight and hirsutism?

Hirsute women are more likely to be obese than non-hirsute women. Thus weight loss must be a priority in treating overweight women with hirsutism.

How would you investigate a patient with suspected POCD?

- Ovarian ultrasound is the most accurate investigation; typically it shows thickened capsules, multiple 3–5 mm cysts and a hyperechogenic stroma.
- Biochemistry:
  Total testosterone levels may be normal, but free androgens are raised.
  Sex-hormone-binding globulin is low.
  LH : FSH ratio is raised, usually greater than 2 : 1, but FSH is low or normal.
  Mild hyperprolactinaemia is common and rarely exceeds $1500\,mUl^{-1}$.

References

Adams, J, Polson, DW & Franks, S (1986) Prevalence of polycystic ovaries in women with anovulation and idiopathic hirsutism. *Br Med J* **293**: 355.
Conway, GS & Jacobs, HS (1990) Hirsutism. *Br Med J* **301**: 619.

Case 143	Acanthosis Nigricans

Instruction

Do a general examination.

Salient features

- Black, velvety overgrowth seen in the axillae, neck, umbilicus, nipples, groins or facial skin.
- Look for the following signs:
  Tripe palms (roughness of the palmar and plantar skin).
  Filiform growths around the face and mouth, and over the tongue.
- Tell the examiner that you would like to investigate for underlying malignancy, in particular adenocarcinoma of the stomach.

Questions

With which other conditions is acanthosis nigricans associated?

- Lymphoma.
- Diabetes mellitus associated with insulin resistance in young children.
- Cushing's syndrome.
- Acromegaly.
- Stein–Leventhal syndrome.

What is the relationship between the course of the skin lesion and the underlying malignancy?

The acanthosis nigricans may precede the neoplasm by more than 5 years. In about two thirds of cases the course parallels that of the tumour, including remission with cure.

Mention some cutaneous manifestations of visceral malignancy.

- Dermatomyositis.
- Migratory thrombophlebitis.
- Ichthyosis.
- Paget's disease of the nipple.

| Case 144 | Lipoatrophy |

Instruction

Look at this patient.
Look here (the examiner pointing at the patient's thighs).

Salient features

- Atrophy of the subcutaneous fat.
- Tell the examiner that you would like to know whether or not the patient is on insulin for diabetes.

Questions

In which other conditions is lipoatrophy seen?

- Localised scleroderma.
- Morphoea.

- Chronic relapsing panniculitis on healing.
- Mesangiocapillary glomerular nephritis.

What advice would you give this patient on insulin?

The insulin should be changed to a more purified form and the patient should rotate the sites of injection.

Case 145	Lupus Pernio

Instruction

Look at this patient's face.

Salient features

- Reddish blue or violaceous plaques on the nose, cheeks, ears and fingers with telangiectasia over and around the plaques.

- Tell the examiner that you would like to do a CXR for hilar lymphadenopathy.

Questions

What is the differential diagnosis of such a lesion?

- Rhinophyma.
- Lupus vulgaris.
- Leprosy.

What are the cutaneous manifestions of sarcoid?

- Erythema nodosum.
- Micropapular sarcoid.

- Scar infiltration.
- Sarcoid plaques of limbs, shoulders, buttocks, thighs.

How may sarcoid present?

- Acute sarcoidosis usually presents in the third decade characterised by erythema nodosum, parotid enlargement and hilar lymphadenopathy.
- Chronic sarcoidosis usually presents in the fifth decade with an insidious onset characterised by fatigue, dyspnoea, arthralgia and lupus pernio. Bone cysts are another feature.

How would you investigate such a patient?

- CXR.
- Slit lamp examination of the eyes.
- Kveim's test (the antigen is cultured in human spleen).
- Mantoux test.
- Serum-angiotensin-converting enzyme test.
- Serum calcium levels.
- Gallium-67 scan.
- Bronchoalveolar lavage.
- Histological confirmation: transbronchial lung biopsy; biopsy of lymph node, skin, liver, gums, minor salivary glands.

What is the prognosis and treatment of sarcoidosis?

- Acute sarcoidosis usually regresses spontaneously within 2 years and does not recur; it may not require treatment.
- Chronic sarcoidosis may require systemic corticosteroids in order to prevent serious disability and even death from respiratory failure.

What are the specific indications for systemic steroids in sarcoidosis?

- Progressive deterioration in lung function, particularly transfer factor and vital capacity. Serial evaluation should be performed every 2 months initially, gradually increasing the intervals between follow-ups to about 4–5 months; patients should be followed up for at least 2 years after steroids are stopped.
- CNS involvement.
- Hypercalcaemia.
- Severe ocular disease.

What are the ocular manifestations of sarcoidosis?

- Anterior uveitis, seen in about 5% of all cases:
    Acute.
    Chronic – mutton fat keratic precipitates, iris nodules.

- Retinal vasculitis, neovascularisation.
- Vitreous opacities.
- Choroidal granulomata.
- Optic nerve granuloma.

What is Löfgren's syndrome?

Erythema nodosum and hilar adenopathy in a patient with sarcoidosis.

MA Kveim (b.1892), Norwegian pathologist.
S Löfgren, Swedish physician.
D Geraint James, contemporary Professor of Medicine, Royal Free Hospital, London; his chief interest is sarcoidosis.

References

James, DG & Jones Williams, W (1984) *Sarcoidosis and other Granulomatous Disorders*. Philadelphia: WB Saunders.
Spalton, DJ & Sanders, MD (1981) Fundus changes in histologically confirmed sarcoidosis. *Br J Ophthalmol* **65**: 348–358.

Case 146	Xanthelasma

Instruction

Examine this patient's eyes.

Salient features

- Xanthelasmata (flat yellow nodules or plaques) seen around both eyes, particularly on the inner canthus.
- Look for the following signs:
    Corneal arcus.

Jaundice, generalised pigmentation, scratch marks (primary biliary cirrhosis).
Tendon xanthomas.
Palmar xanthomata.
- Tell the examiner that you would like to check the following:
  Urine sugar.
  Blood pressure.

Remember that blood lipids can often be normal in such patients.

Questions

In which conditions is xanthelasma seen?

Those in which there is an increase in serum cholesterol:
- Type IIb hyperlipidaemia – increase in cholesterol and triglycerides.
- Type IIa hyperlipidaemia – increase in cholesterol only.
- Type III hyperlipidaemia – equal increase in cholesterol and triglycerides.

Mention a few secondary causes of hyperlipidaemia.

Diabetes mellitus, hypothyroidism, nephrotic syndrome, cholestatic jaundice, excess alcohol intake, oral contraceptives.

How would you manage a patient with hyperlipidaemia?

- Life style advice.
- Dietary modification (usually adequate for those whose cholesterol is in the range $6.5–8\,\mathrm{mmol\,l^{-1}}$).
- Avoidance of alcohol, smoking, oestrogens and thiazides.
- Exercise.
- Control of hypertension and diabetes.
- Lipid-lowering drugs.

Mention a few lipid-lowering drugs.

- Ion exchange resin:
  Cholestyramine.
- Fibrates:
  Bezafibrate.
  Gemfibrizil.
- Human menopausal gonadotrophin.
- (HMG) coenzyme A (CoA) reductase inhibitors:
  Simvastatin.
  Lovastatin.

- Nicotinic acid derivatives:
  Nicotinic acid.
  Probucol.

Case 147	Necrobiosis Lipodica Diabeticorum

Instruction

Examine this patient's legs.
Examine this patient's back.

Salient features

- Usually in females.
- Sharply demarcated oval plaques seen on the shin, arms or back.
- The plaques have a shiny surface with yellow waxy centres and brownish red margins with surrounding telangiectasia.

- Tell the examiner that you would like to check the urine for sugar.

Questions

What is the histology?

Collagen degeneration surrounded by epitheloid and giant cells.

What may complicate it?

Ulceration of the plaque.

What treatment is available for such lesions?

- Good diabetic control.
- Local steroids.
- Excision and skin grafting.

What other skin lesions are usually seen on the shins?

- Erythema nodosum.
- Pretibial myxoedema.
- Diabetic dermopathy.
- Erythema ab igne.
- Livedo reticularis.

What are the other skin lesions seen in diabetics?

- Granuloma annulare.
- Carbuncles.
- Vitiligo.
- Fat atrophy and hypertrophy.
- Leg ulcers and gangrene.
- Acanthosis nigricans.
- Vulval candidiasis.

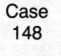

Case 148   Radiotherapy Marks

Instruction

Look at these patients' chests.

Salient features

Patient 1:
- Telangiectasia over the chest wall.
- There may be a unilateral mastectomy.
This patient had radiotherapy for breast cancer in the past.

Patient 2:
- India ink marks over the chest.
- Localised erythema in the same region.
This patient is undergoing radiotherapy treatment.

Questions

In which conditions is radiotherapy beneficial?

- Malignant conditions: intracranial tumours, Hodgkin's disease, meningeal carcinomatosis, pathological fractures secondary to malignancy, spinal cord compression, superior vena caval obstruction, cancer pain, dysphagia of terminal illness, head and neck cancers, pituitary tumours, ovarian tumours, upper airway obstruction, pericardial tamponade secondary to malignant pericardial tumours.
- Nonmalignant conditions:
  Exophthalmos.
  Rheumatoid arthritis (total lymphoid irradiation is an experimental therapeutic procedure).
  Ankylosing spondylitis (spinal irradiation is no longer used due to the risk of haematological malignancy; however, local external irradiation of an involved peripheral joint or an injected radiation synovectomy can be valuable in ameliorating pain and allowing mobility).

References

Horwich, A (1992) Current issues in cancer: radiotherapy update. *Br Med J* **304:** 1554.

Case 149	Tendon Xanthomata

Instruction

Look at this patient's hands.

Salient features

- Tendon xanthomata seen on the extensor tendons and becoming more prominent when the patient clenches his or her fist.
- Look at other tendons, i.e. the patellar and Achilles tendons.
- Look at the eyes for xanthelasmata and corneal arcus.
- Tell the examiner that you would like to check fasting lipids, in particular for cholesterol elevation.

Questions

In which condition are these seen?

Familial hypercholesterolemia, an autosomal dominant trait with an excess of low-density lipoprotein (LDL) or betalipoprotein in the blood. It occurs in 1 in 200–500 of the population.

What is the basic defect?

Goldstein and Brown, in 1975, showed that this condition was due to defect or deficiency in LDL cell receptors. They were awarded the Nobel prize for their work.

At what age do these patients manifest?

Homozygotes usually have xanthomata at birth or as children. They have a predisposition to ischaemic heart disease which usually results in death before the age of 30. About 50% of heterozygotes also present by the same age.

James Scott, contemporary Professor and Chairman of the Department of Medicine at the Hammersmith Hospital, London, is a physician, biochemist and molecular biologist. He has made a considerable contribution to cholesterol research.

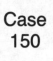

Case 150 — Eruptive Xanthomata

Instruction

Examine this patient's skin.
This uncontrolled diabetic has developed this profuse eruption; what are these lesions?

Salient features

- Multiple, itchy, red-yellow vesicles or nodules which are seen over extensor surfaces, i.e. buttocks, back, knees and elbows.
- Tell the examiner that you would like to examine the fundus for lipaemia retinalis.
- Tell the examiner that you would like to check urine for sugar and do a lipid profile.

Remember that eruptive xanthomata signify triglyceridaemia.

Questions

In which conditions are eruptive xanthoma seen?

- Type IV hyperlipidaemia.
  Familial hypertriglyceridaemia.
  Lipoprotein lipase deficiency.
  Apolipoprotein CII deficiency.
- Type I hyperlipidaemia – chylomicronaemia.
- Type V hyperlipidaemia – increased triglycerides and chylomicrons.

Case 151	Palmar Xanthomata

Instruction

Examine this patient's hands.

Salient features

- Yellowish-orange discolorations over the palmar and digital creases.
- Look for the following signs:
  Xanthelasmata around the eyes.
  Tuboeruptive xanthomata around the elbows and knees.
- Tell the examiner that this patient probably has a type III hyperlipidaemia.

Note. A more generalised form may be associated with monoclonal gammopathy of myeloma or lymphoma.

Questions

How would you classify hyperlipidaemia?

Fredrickson' classification, depending on laboratory findings:

- Type I: elevated chylomicrons and triglycerides, normal cholesterol (pancreatitis, eruptive xanthomas and lipaemia retinalis).
- Type IIa: elevated LDL and cholesterol, normal triglycerides (premature coronary artery disease, tendon xanthomas and arcus cornea).
- Type IIb: elevated LDL, very-low-density lipoprotein (VLDL), cholesterol and triglycerides (premature coronary artery disease).
- Type III: elevated β-VLDL (cholesterol-rich) remnants, cholesterol and triglycerides (premature coronary artery disease, peripheral vascular disease, palmar and tuberous xanthomas).
- Type IV: elevated VLDL and triglycerides, normal cholesterol (premature coronary artery disease – in some forms; risk of developing chylomicronaemia syndrome).
- Type V: elevated chylomicrons, VLDL, cholestrol and triglycerides (pancreatitis, eruptive xanthomas, lipaemia retinalis).

What are causes of secondary hyperlipidaemia?

Elevated cholesterol:

- Biliary cirrhosis.
- Hypothyroidism.
- Nephrotic syndrome.

Elevated triglycerides:

- Alcohol abuse.
- Diabetes.
- Renal failure.
- Oral contraceptives.

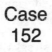
Case 152   Pseudoxanthoma Elasticum

Instruction

Look at this patient's fundus (*Patient 1*).

Salient features

- Fundus shows angioid streaks, i.e. linear grey or dark red streaks with irregular edges which lie beneath the retinal vessels (roughly 50% of patients with angioid streaks have pseudoxanthoma elasticum whereas 85% of patients with pseudoxanthoma have angioid streaks).

- Look at the neck, antecubital fossae, axillae, groins and periumbilical region for loose 'chicken skin' appearance of skin.

Instruction

Look at this patient (*Patient 2*).

Salient features

- Small yellow papules arranged in a linear or reticulate pattern in plaques on the neck, axillae cubital fossae, periumbilical region and groin.
- Tell the examiner that you would like to examine the fundus.

Questions

In which other conditions are angioid streaks seen?

Ehlers–Danlos syndrome, Paget's disease, sickle cell disease.

What are angioid streaks caused by?

Abnormal elastic tissue in the Bruch's membrane of the retina.

Which fundal finding is virtually pathognomonic of pseudoxanthoma elasticum?

'Leopard skin spotting' changes which consist of yellowish mottling of the posterior pole temporal to the macula. These may antedate angioid streaks.

What is the triad of pseudoxanthoma elasticum, angioid streaks and vascular abnormalities known as?

Groenblad–Strandberg syndrome.

What are the cardiovascular manifestations of this condition?

- Mitral valve prolapse.
- Accelerated atherosclerosis.
- Renovascular hypertension.
- Premature coronary artery disease.
- Peripheral vascular disease.

What are the gastrointestinal manifestations of this disease?

Gastrointestinal haemorrhage, particularly during the first decade.

What are the causes of visual loss?

Macular involvement by a streak; disciform scarring secondary to choroidal haemorrhage, or traumatic macular haemorrhage.

KWL Bruch (1819–1884), Professor of Anatomy at Giessen, Germany.
EE Groenblad, Swedish ophthalmologist.

J Strandberg, Swedish dermatologist.
TL Terry (1899–1946) Head of Ophthalmology at Harvard University, described angioid streaks in Paget's disease.

References

Clarkson, JG & Altman, RD (1982) Angioid streaks. *Surv Ophthalmol* **26**: 235–246.
Lebwohl, MG, Distefano, D, Prioleau, PG et al (1982) Pseudoxanthoma elasticum and mitral valve prolapse. *N Engl J Med* **307**: 228–231.

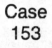 **Rosacea**

Case 153

Instruction

Look at this patient.

Salient features

- Red patch with telangiectasia, papules and pustules overlying the flush areas of the face, i.e. cheeks, chin and nose. (The papules and pustules distinguish it from the rash of SLE.)
- Comment on the following:
    Rhinophyma (irregular thickening of the skin of the nose with enlarged follicular orifices).
    Blepharitis, conjunctivitis.

Questions

How would you manage such a patient?

- Avoid factors which provoke facial flushing.
- Tetracycline or metronidazole.

- Hydrocortisone cream.
- Retinoids – in resistant disease.
- Surgical removal for rhinophyma.

| Case 154 | Dermatitis Herpetiformis |

Instruction

Look at this patient's skin.

Salient features

- Dry itchy vesicles on both elbows.
- Look for similar lesions on the scalp, face, neck, shoulders, buttocks, knees and calves.
- Tell the examiner that you would like to take a history of diarrhoea and gluten intolerance.

Questions

From which other itchy skin disorder should dermatitis herpetiformis be differentiated?

Scabies.

How would you investigate such a patient?

- Skin biopsy: subepidermal vesicle with a neutrophilic infiltrate. Immunofluorescence demonstrates granular dermal papillary IgA deposits.
- Jejunal biopsy: patchy abnormality showing subtotal villous atrophy with increased lymphocyte infiltration in the epithelium.

- Therapeutic test: dapsone dramatically reduces itching in 72 hours, often providing confirmation before the biopsy result is available.
- HLA-B8 is positive in more than 80% of the patients.

How would you treat such a patient?

- Gluten restriction.
- Dapsone or sulphapyridine – neither drug should be given to a patient with glucose-6-phosphate deficiency. Treatment is lifelong; there is usually a rapid relapse if the drug is stopped.

In which foods is gluten found?

Wheat, barley, rye and possibly oats (rice and maize are permitted in these patients).

What are the benefits of a gluten-free diet?

It gradually improves skin lesions, improves any associated manifestations of malabsorptive enteropathy and may reduce the late risk of intestinal lymphoma.

Case 155 Hairy Leucoplakia

Instruction

Look at this patient's tongue.

Salient features

- Shaggy, hairy, white lesions on the lateral margins of the tongue.
- Tell the examiner that you would like to know whether or not the patient is infected by the HIV virus.

Questions

What is the cause for this lesion?

Cytomegalovirus has been implicated as it has been demonstrated in the upper spinous layers of the epithelium.

What are the histological features of this condition?

- Hyperkeratosis.
- Hyperplasia and ballooning of prickle cells.
- Depletion of Langerhans' cells.

How would you treat this condition?

Treatment is seldom indicated, but ganciclovir may be helpful if treatment is needed.

P Langerhans (1847–1888), German pathologist and dermatologist.

References

Editorial (1989) Oral hairy leucoplakia. *Lancet* **2**: 1195.

Case 156   Kaposi's Sarcoma

Instruction

Look at this skin lesion.

Salient features

- Plum-coloured violet plaques, either solitary or in crops, on the limbs, mouth, tip of the nose and palate.

- Tell the examiner that you would like to check HIV antibody titres.

Questions

What are the varieties of Kaposi's sarcoma?

- African variety: violaceous skin plaques, black under Negroid skin; an aggressive invasive tumour which is ultimately fatal.
- Classic Kaposi's: initially described in Jews; indolent; found on the legs of elderly men; confined to the skin and may be present for decades; not fatal.
- Associated with sexually transmitted AIDS (as above).

How would you manage such patients?

In Kaposi's sarcoma due to AIDS radiotherapy or chemotherapy may help; however, the majority of them relapse. Prognosis is poor.

Moritz Kaposi (1837–1902) in 1872 described these as 'idiopathic multiple pigmented sarcoma'. He also described the rash in SLE as 'butterfly rash' in 1875.

| Case 157 | Peutz–Jeghers Syndrome |

Instruction

Look at this patient's face.

Salient features

- Pigmented freckles around the lips.
- Look in the mouth for similar pigmentation and anaemia.
- Tell the examiner that you would like to take a history of the following:

Pain in the abdomen due to intestinal intussusception.
Gastrointestinal haemorrhage in the upper gastrointestinal tract, or rectal bleeding.
Family involvement (autosomal dominant).

Questions

What are the types of colonic polyps?

- Tubular adenomas: over 60% are in the rectosigmoid colon and may cause bleeding or obstruction. The risk of malignancy correlates with the size. The tubular adenoma is removed endoscopically. Follow-up surveillance is by colonoscopy every 2 years.
- Villous adenomas are usually found in the left colon and have a high risk of malignancy. Polyps larger than 2 cm have a 50% risk of malignancy. They may present with hypokalaemia due to potassium loss in the stools. They are removed by colonoscopic resection.
- Hyperplastic polyps are benign and rarely undergo malignant change. It is usually detected as an incidental finding at colonoscopy.

What polyposis syndromes do you know?

- Familial adenomatous polyposis (FAP): autosomal dominant inheritance (there is an abnormality of chromosome 5) with several thousand polyps throughout the colon. The potential for malignant change is 100% by the age of 40 and hence all patients ought to have prophylactic colectomy before the age of 30. All relatives ought to be screened from the age of 12.
- Gardner's syndrome: a variant of FAP in which additional features are soft tissue tumours (osteomas, lipomas, dermoid tumours) and pigmentation of the fundi.
- Juvenile polyps: an autosomal dominant condition occurring in children and teenagers. It may cause gastrointestinal bleeds, abdominal pain, diarrhoea and intussusception. There is an increased incidence of malignant change in the interspersed adenomatous polyps.
- Peutz–Jeghers syndrome: characterised by mucocutaneous melanosis with gastrointestinal hamartomas. The inheritance is autosomal dominant. The intestinal polyps may give rise to haematemesis, melaena or rectal bleeding, anaemia or intussusception depending on their location. These polyps are usually found in the ileum and jejunum and they rarely undergo malignant change.
- Cronkhite–Canada syndrome: sporadic; colonic, small bowel or gastric polyps associated with ectodermal changes such as hyperpigmentation, nail atrophy and alopecia.

- Turcot syndrome: autosomal recessive; colorectal polyps associated with CNS tumours.
- Cowden's disease: autosomal dominant; multiple gastrointestinal hamartomas with warty papules on the mucosa and skin malformations.

This condition was originally described by JL Peutz of Holland in 1921 and rediscovered by HJ Jeghers et al of USA in 1949.
EJ Gardner (b.1909), US geneticist and Professor of Zoology at Utah University.
J Turcot, Canadian Surgeon.
LW Cronkhite, physician, Massachusetts General Hospital.
Wilma J Canada, US radiologist.

References

Bulow, S (1984) Colrectal polyposis syndromes. *Scand J Gastroenterol* **19:** 289.
Gardner, EJ, Burt, RW & Freston, JW (1980) Gastrointestinal polyposis: syndromes and genetic mechanisms. *West J Med* **132:** 488.

| Case 158 | Pyoderma Gangrenosum |

Instruction

Look at this patient's skin.

Salient features

- Necrotic ulcer with purplish overhanging edges, usually seen on the lower limbs or trunk.
- Tell the examiner that you would like to take a history of the following:
  Diarrhoea (inflammatory bowel disease).
  Joint pains (rheumatoid arthritis).

Questions

In which conditions can pyoderma gangrenosum be seen?

- Ulcerative colitis.
- Crohn's disease.
- Chronic active hepatitis.
- Rheumatoid arthritis.
- Acute and chronic myeloid leukaemia.
- Polycythaemia rubra vera.
- Multiple myeloma.
- IgA monoclonal gammopathy.
- No cause in 50% of cases.

How would you manage these lesions?

- High-dose steroids.
- Intralesional steriods.
- Some regress with treatment of the underlying cause.

| Case 159 | Sturge–Weber Syndrome |

Instruction

Look at this patient's face.

Salient features

- A port wine stain is present on the face in the distribution of the first and second divisions of the trigeminal nerve.
- Hypertrophy of the involved area of the face.
- Look for haemangiomas of the episclera and the iris.
- Tell the examiner that you would like to proceed as follows:

Examine the fundus for unilateral choroidal haemangioma.
Take a history of seizures.
Do a skull X-ray for intracranial 'tramline' calcification, particularly in the parieto occipital lobe.

Questions

What is the inheritance in such patients?

This is the only syndrome of the phacomatoses that does not have a hereditary tendency. It occurs sporadically and has no sexual predilection.

What are the neurological manifestations in such patients?

Jacksonian epilepsy, contralateral hemianopia, hemisensory disturbance, hemiparesis and hemianopia, low IQ.

What other ocular manifestations do you know?

Glaucoma (in 30% of cases), buphthalmos (large eye), optic atrophy.

How would you treat such a patient?

Treatment is aimed at pharmacological control of seizures. The patient should be referred to the ophthalmologist for management of increased intraocular pressure or choroidal angioma.

Siegfried Kalischer, a German pathologist, described postmortem findings in a case as early as in 1901.
William A Sturge (1850–1919), a London physician, described this condition in 1879. He was attached to the Royal Free Hospital, London, and founded the Society of Prehistoric Archaeology in East Anglia.
Frederick Parkes Weber (1863–1962), a London physician, was the first to describe the radiological appearances in this condition. Two other syndromes to which Weber's name is attached are Weber–Christian disease (relapsing, febrile, nodular, nonsuppurative panniculitis) and Osler–Rendu–Weber syndrome (hereditary haemorrhagic telangiectasia).

Case 160	**Acne Vulgaris**

Instruction

Look at this patient.

Salient features

- Comedones, or blackheads, usually on the chin, face, shoulders and upper chest (due to plugging of hair follicles by keratin).
- Whiteheads (i.e. distended sebaceous glands without a pore).
- Cysts (larger, deeper masses of retained sebum).
- Greasy skin.
- There may be associated scarring.

- Tell the examiner that you would like to take a history of the following:
  Steroid ingestion.
  Isoniazid ingestion.
  Occupational exposure to oils (oil-induced acne).

Questions

How would you manage acne?

- Wash affected parts with soap not more than twice a day.
- Avoid steaming, saunas, Turkish baths.
- Topical therapy: sulphur, benzyl peroxide, retinoic acid.
- Systemic therapy: tetracycline, erythromycin, isotretinoin.

Have you heard of acne fulminans?

It is a rare variant, seen exclusively in adolescent boys. The lesions eventually become necrotic and form haemorrhagic crusts, causing disfiguring and scarring. There may be associated systemic features such as fever, malaise, arthralgia, arthritis and vasculitis.

What do you know about acne conglobata?

It is seen in tall Caucasian males with cystic skin lesions and multiple abscess formation. It rarely regresses.

| Case 161 | Mycosis Fungoides (Cutaneous T-Cell Lymphoma) |

Instruction

Look at this patient's skin.

Salient features

- Itchy, brownish-red plaques on the hips, buttocks and interscapular region, usually seen in the fifth and sixth decade.
- Tell the examiner that it may also involve the lymph nodes and viscera.

Questions

How would you confirm the diagnosis?

Skin biopsy, to detect Pautrier's microabscesses, atypical cells in nests in the epidermis, atypical mononuclear cell infiltrates, large hyperchromatic cells with irregular nuclei, the 'mycosis cells'.

What is the prognosis?

Very slow progression of skin lesions with eventual tumour formation and systemic dissemination of lymphoma. In most patients this process takes several decades.

What is the differential diagnosis?

Psoriasis.

How would you treat this patient?

Treatment is palliative, using steroids, chemotherapeutic agents and electron beam therapy.

What are the stages of cutaneous T-cell lymphoma?

- Stage I: eczematoid or psoriasiform erythematous lesions.
- Stage II: infiltrated plaques.

- Stage III: nodules, ulcers, tumours.
- Stage IV: lymph node involvement with or without systemic dissemination.

Have you heard of Sézary's syndrome?

It is an erythrodermatous variant of mycosis fungoides characterised by extensive erythroderma, lymphadenopathy and large mononuclear cells (Sézary cells) in the skin and the blood.

Jean Louis M Alibert, a French dermatologist, first described this condition in 1806.
A Sézary (1880–1956), French dermatologist.

| Case 162 | Urticaria Pigmentosa |

Instruction

Look at this patient's skin.

Salient features

- Itchy, reddish-brown macules and papules.
- Telangiectasia.

- Look for hepatosplenomegaly.
- Tell the examiner that you would like to take a history of the following:
    Urticaria with pruritus on trauma, rubbing or heat – Darier's sign.
    Headache.
    Diarrhoea.
    Itching.

Questions

What do you know about urticaria pigmentosa?

It is the cutaneous manifestation of systemic mastocytosis.

What do you know about systemic mastocytosis?

It is a condition characterised by mast cell hyperplasia which in most cases is neither clonal nor neoplastic. It can occur at any age and is slightly more common in men. Four forms have been recognised:

- Indolent form: does not alter life expectancy and constitutes the majority of the cases.
- Associated with frank leukaemia or dysmyelopoiesis: the prognosis is determined by the underlying haematological disorder.
- Aggressive form: the prognosis is determined by the extent of organ involvement.
- Mast cell leukaemia: rare, invariably fatal.

How would you manage such patients?

- H_1 blocker – for flushing and itch (e.g. chlormethiazole).
- H_2 blocker – for gastric and duodenal manifestations (e.g. ranitidine, cimetidine).
- Oral sodium cromoglycate for diarrhoea and abdominal pain.
- NSAID for flushing not responsive to antihistamines.

JF Darier (1856–1938), French dermatologist.

MISCELLANEOUS

Examination of Feet

1. Inspection
   - Comment on deformity: hallux valgus, pes cavus.
   - Skin: comment on the colour, ulcers and gangrene, hair loss (remember that this is not a reliable sign of ischaemia).
   - Joint: comment on the swelling, e.g. ankle joint, first meta-tarsophalangeal joint in gout.

2. Palpation
   - Ask the patient if the foot is sore.
   - Feel for temperature difference between the two feet.
   - Pulses: dorsalis pedis and posterior tibials (compare with the other side).
   - Sensation: check light touch, pain and joint sensation.
   - Check the plantar response and the ankle jerk.

| Case 163 | Diabetic Foot |

Instruction

Examine this patient's legs.
Examine this patient's feet.

Salient features

Neuropathic foot:

- Dry, warm and pink with palpable pulses.
- Impaired deep tendon reflexes.
- Reduced pinprick, light touch and vibration sensation.

Ischaemic foot:

- Skin is shiny and atrophic with sparse hair.
- The foot is cool and peripheral pulses are absent.
- Tell the examiner that you would like to check all peripheral pulses.

Neuropathic and ischaemic foot present together:

- Ulcer on the foot with callosities at pressure points.
- Loss of arch of foot.
- Stocking distribution of sensory loss of all modalities.
- Loss of dorsalis pedis and/or posterior tibial pulsations.
- Tell the examiner that you would like to check the urine for sugar.

- When asked to examine the feet remember that the common conditions affecting the feet are diabetes and atherosclerosis – pay particular attention to the pulses and skin.

Questions

What are the types of diabetic foot?

- Neuropathic foot.
- Ischaemic foot.

Note. Features of both types often occur together.

Mention a few conditions in which neuropathic ulcers are seen.

- Progressive sensory neuropathy.
- Tabes dorsalis.
- Leprosy.
- Amyloidosis.
- Porphyria.

How would you manage this patient?

- X-ray of the foot.
- Antibiotics.
- Removal of necrotic tissue.
- Remove weight bearing and friction from ulcerated areas – appropriate footwear such as moulded insoles or plaster cast, or crutches to avoid weight bearing.

- Control hyperglycaemia.
- Chiropody.
- Surgical opinion and arteriography if reconstructive vascular surgery is to be considered.

What would you monitor in a diabetic at annual review?

- Eyes: visual acuity, fundoscopy.
- Sensory system: touch, pinprick and vibration sense.
- Deep tendon reflexes.
- Cardiovascular system: blood pressure, peripheral pulses.
- Biochemistry: urine and blood sugar, albumin, glycosylated haemoglobin, creatinine.

References

Elkeles, RS & Wolfe, JHN (1991) ABC of vascular diseases: the diabetic foot. *Br Med J* **303:** 1053.

Case 164	Swollen Leg

Instruction

Look at this patient's leg.

Salient features

Patient 1 has *deep vein thrombosis.*

- Painful calf.
- Redness.
- Engorged superficial veins.
- Unilateral swollen leg with pitting oedema.

- Pain on the calf on dorsiflexion of the foot – Homan's sign (not a diagnostic sign).

- Check for pitting oedema on both sides (look at the patient's eyes while eliciting this sign, to ensure that you are not hurting the patient).
- Compare the temperature of both the legs (use the dorsum of your fingers to elicit this sign).
- Check the arterial pulses in the leg.
- Tell the examiner that you would like to know whether the swelling is acute or chonic.
- Remember to collect your thoughts when asked to examine the legs – do not rush in to grab the patient's legs.

Questions

What are the complications of a deep vein thrombosis?

- Pulmonary embolism.
- Venous gangrene.
- Pain, particularly in iliofemoral thrombosis.

What are the predisposing factors for venous thrombosis?

- Surgery.
- Prolonged immobility.
- Old age.
- Obesity.
- Malignancy.
- Varicose veins.
- Pregnancy.
- Oral contraceptives.

How would you investigate a patient with suspected deep vein thrombosis?

As clinical diagnosis is unreliable it is essential to perform the following investigations to assess the extent of thrombosis:

- Duplex ultrasound scanning and Doppler studies.
- Venogram – by injecting contrast into one of leg veins.

What is the risk of pulmonary embolism in below-knee thrombi?

The risk in such cases is low and many physicians refrain from anticoagulating these patients.

How would you treat these patients?

- Pain relief.
- Elastic support stockings.
- The main aim is to prevent pulmonary emboli and all patients with thrombi above the knee must be anticoagulated:
  Intravenous heparin for 48 hours.
  Oral anticoagulants for at least 3 months.

Salient features

Patient 2 has *cellulitis*.

- Red, inflamed leg with a definite demarcation of the erythematous area.
- Oedema.
- Increased temperature.

- Examine the peripheral pulses.
- Ask the patient whether he or she had fever.
- Look for superficial ulcers.

Questions

How would you manage such a patient?

- Blood cultures.
- Intravenous antibiotics.
- Pain relief and antipyretics.
- Surgical referral.

What are the causes of bilateral swollen legs?

- Cardiac failure.
- Renal failure.
- Hypoproteinaemia resulting from cirrhosis or nephrotic syndrome.

What are the causes of an acutely swollen leg?

- Deep vein thrombosis.
- Cellulitis.
- Arterial occlusion.
- Trauma.
- Arthritis.

What are the causes of a chronically swollen leg?

- Venous causes: varicose veins, postphlebitic limb.
- Lymphoedema: Milroy's disease, filariasis (in the tropics).
- Congenital.

J Homan (1877–1954) was an American surgeon who worked at Johns Hopkins Hospital with Cushing, initially on experimental hypophysectomy and later on vascular disease.
WF Milroy (1855–1942) described familial lymphoedema of the legs in 1892.

References

Reilly, DT & Wolfe, JHN (1991) ABC of vascular diseases: the swollen leg. *Br Med J* **303:** 1462.

| Case 165 | Clubbing |

Instruction

Examine this patient's hands.

Salient features

- Increased curvature of the nails, obliteration of the angle of the nail (when in doubt, approximate the dorsal aspects of fingers of both hands which are flexed at the interphalangeal joints).
- The nails may have a drumstick appearance.
- Look for the following signs:
    Fluctuation at the nail bed.
    Palpate the wrist joints for tenderness hypertrophic pulmonary osteoarthropathy (HPOA).
    Nicotine (tar) staining of fingers.

Central cyanosis.
Clubbing of the toes.
- Tell the examiner that you would like to examine the following areas:
    Chest (bronchogenic carcinoma; fibrosing alveolitis; suppurative lung disease such as bronchiectasis, lung abscess and empyema; mesothelioma).
    Heart (infective endocarditis, cyanotic heart disease).
    Gastrointestinal tract (ulcerative colitis, Crohn's disease).
    Thyroid (thyroid acropachy).
- If an underlying cause is obvious, ask for a family history in order to confirm a hereditary cause of clubbing.

Questions

What are the mechanisms for clubbing?

- Increased blood flow in clubbed fingers duc to vasodilatation rather than hyperplasia of vessels in the nail bed. The nature of the vaso-dilator is unclear and many contenders, such as ferritin, bradykinin, prostaglandin and 5-hydroxytryptamine (5-HT), have been impli-cated. The vasodilator is probably inactivated in the lung in normal persons but when this inactivation is defective or in the presence of a right-to-left shunt clubbing occurs.
- Increased growth hormone (GH) in disease states causes excessive growth of cellular tissue in the nail bed.
- Clubbing occurs whenever organs supplied by the vagus are affected. It has been shown that, in bronchogenic carcinoma, vagotomy causes reversal of clubbing.
- Tumour necrosis factor has been implicated.
- Megakaryocytes and clumps of platelets may preferentially stream into blood vessels of the digits and release platelet-derived growth factor. The resulting increased capillary permeability, fibroblastic activity and arterial smooth muscle hyperplasia could cause clubbing.

References

Anonymous (1990) Is clubbing a growth disorder? *Lancet* **336**: 848.
Dickinson, CJ & Martin, JF (1987) Megakaryocytes and platelet clumps as the cause of finger clubbing. *Lancet* **ii**: 1434–1435.

Case 166	Dupuytren's Contracture

Instruction

Look at this patient's hands.

Salient features

- Thickening of the palmar fascia, particularly along the medial aspect. (Feel for thickening before you comment on it.)
- Tell the examiner that you would like to check the feet for contracture of the plantar fascia.

Questions

With which other conditions is Dupuytren's contracture associated?

- Alcoholism.
- Chronic antiepileptic therapy.
- Thickening of the corpora cavernosa of the penis (Peyronie's disease).
- Garrod's knuckle pads.
- Retroperitoneal fibrosis.

Baron Guillaume Dupuytren (1777–1835), Surgeon-in-Chief, Hôtel-Dieu, Paris, is reported to have been the first to achieve successful removal of the lower jaw.
Sir AE Garrod (1857–1936), London physician at St Bartholomew's Hospital, succeeded Osler as Regius Professor at Oxford.
F de la Peyronie (1678–1747), French surgeon who influenced Louis XVI in his decision to issue an ordinance banning barbers from practising surgery.

Case 167 | Cataracts

Instruction

Examine this patient's eyes.

Salient features

- Bilateral cataracts (shine light obliquely across the lens).
- Tell the examiner that you would like to proceed as follows:
  Check urine for sugar.
  Take a drug history – steroids, chloroquine.

Questions

Mention a few causes of cataracts.

- *Common causes:*
  Old age (look for arcus senilis).
  Diabetes mellitus.
- *Uncommon causes:*
  Trauma.
  Cushing's syndrome.
  Dystrophia myotonica.
  Congenital rubella.
  Drugs (chloroquine, steroids, phenothiazines, chlorambucil, busulphan).
  Hypoparathyroidism.

How are cataracts treated?

Cataract extraction is performed by removing the lens nucleus and cortex from within the lens capsule. In most adults, a plastic lens is implanted within the capsule.

Case 168	Anaemia

Instruction

Would you like to ask this anaemic patient (*Patient 1*) a few questions?

Salient features

- Ask about the following:
  Blood loss such as bleeding per rectum, melaena, haematemesis, menstrual blood loss.
  Drug history – NSAIDs, phenytoin, chloramphenicol.
  Associated symptoms such as weight loss, shortness of breath, chronic diarrhoea.
  Diet – in vegans, alcoholics, elderly patients.
  Past history of gastrectomy.

Instruction

Would you like to examine this anaemic patient (*Patient 2*)?

Salient features

- Examine the following:
  Nails for koilonychia of iron deficiency anaemia, and (rarely) for clubbing of infective endocarditis.
  Comment on the pallor of the face and conjunctiva, looking for the lemon yellow hue of pernicious anaemia.
  Tongue for glossitis of vitamin B_{12} deficiency.
  Mouth for angular stomatitis of severe malnutrition, and ulcers of neutropenia.
  Lymph nodes in the neck, axillae and groin (secondaries, lymphoproliferative disorders).
  Skin for bruising associated with bone marrow depression seen in leukaemia and aplastic anaemia.
  Abdomen for hepatomegaly, splenomegaly and other masses.
  Legs for ulcers seen in haemoglobinopathies.

- Comment on the ethnic origin (thalassaemia).
- Tell the examiner that you would like to proceed as follows:
  Do a rectal examination and inspect stool for occult blood.
  Do a FBC including a peripheral smear and ESR.

Questions

Mention a few causes of anaemia.

- With a low mean corpuscular volume (MCV):
  Iron deficiency anaemia.
  Thalassemia.
  Sideroblastic anaemia.
- With a high MCV:
  Vitamin B_{12} deficiency (pernicious anaemia, vegans, alcoholics, coeliac disease).
  Folate deficiency (pregnancy, phenytoin, sprue, coeliac disease, malignancy, haemolysis).
  Others: myxoedema, liver disease, alcoholics.
- With a normal MCV:
  Uraemia.
  Malignancy.
  Rheumatoid arthritis.
  Aplastic anaemia (myelofibrosis, chloramphenicol, phenylbutazone, gold, anticancer drugs).

What do you know about the Paterson–Kelly syndrome?

It comprises iron deficiency anaemia and dysphagia due to oesophageal webs in middle-aged women. The clinical significance of this syndrome is uncertain. It is also known as Plummer–Vinson syndrome.

What are the common causes of iron deficiency anaemia?

Occult gastrointestinal bleeding from the following:

- Peptic ulcer.
- Carcinoma located anywhere in the gastrointestinal tract.
- Excessive anticoagulation.
- Hereditary haemorrhagic telangicctasia.
- Angiodysplasia of the colon.

How would you investigate microcytic anaemia?

- FBC.
- Serum ferritin.
- Faecal occult blood.

- Upper gastrointestinal endoscopy.
- Barium enema, colonoscopy.
- International normalised ratio (INR) prothrombin time and platelet count.
- Haemoglobin electrophoresis in susceptible ethnic groups (Asians, Afro-Caribbeans).

How would you investigate macrocytic anaemia?

- Peripheral smear.
- Vitamin B_{12} and red cell folate and serum folate concentrations.
- Serum ferritin, plasma iron and total iron-binding capacity (for associated iron deficiency).
- Schilling test.
- Gastric parietal cell and intrinsic factor antibodies.
- Upper gastrointestinal endoscopy.
- Reticulocyte count (a high MCV could be present when the reticulocyte count is over 50%).
- Bone marrow examination.

RF Schilling (b. 1919), Chairman of the Department of Medicine and haematologist at the University of Wisconsin.

Case 169   Lymphadenopathy

Instruction

Do a general examination.
Examine this patient's neck.

Salient features

As soon as you feel a group of lymph nodes, examine drainage areas for obvious pathology. For example:

- Inguinal lymph nodes: examine the lower limbs and external genitalia.
- Axillary lymph nodes: examine the chest, breasts and upper limbs.
- Upper cervical lymph nodes: examine scalp and mouth, and perform an ear, nose and throat (ENT) examination for nasopharyngeal carcinoma.
- Lower cervical and supraclavicular lymph nodes: examine the thyroid, chest, abdomen for gastric carcinoma (Virchow's nodes), and testis.

- Examine other lymph node areas in a systematic manner:
    Submental, submandibular, deep cervical (upper and lower), occipital, posterior triangle, supraclavicular, axillary, epitrochlear and inguinal.
- Examine the mouth for the following signs:
    Tonsillar lymph nodes.
    Palatal petechiae and pharyngitis (glandular fever).
    Neoplastic tumours or ulcers.
- Tell the examiner that you would like to proceed as follows:
    Examine the abdomen for liver and spleen.
    Examine the chest and do a CXR (for bronchogenic carcinoma, TB).
- Differential diagnosis of generalised lymphadenopathy:
    Lymphomas, chronic lymphatic leukaemia, acute lymphoblastic leukaemia.
    Glandular fever, cytomegalovirus.
    AIDS, toxoplasmosis.
    SLE, rheumatoid arthritis, sarcoid.
    Chronic infections such as TB, secondary syphilis, brucellosis.
    Drugs – phenytoin.

RLK Virchow (1821–1902), successively Professor of Pathology at Würzburg and Berlin. He also described the Virchow cell (lepra cell), Virchow space (perivascular space of Virchow–Robin) and Virchow triad of the pathogenesis of thrombosis.
Thomas Hodgkin (1798–1866), English physician at St Thomas's, London. He was the Curator of the Pathology Museum at Guy's Hospital prior to this.

References

Carde, P (1992) Current issues in cancer: Hodgkin's lymphoma I & II. *Br Med J* **305**: 99, 173.
O'Reilly, SE & Connors, JM (1992) Current issues in cancer: non-hodgkin's lymphoma. *Br Med J* **304**: 1682.

| Case 170 | Chronic Lymphatic Leukaemia |

Instruction

Perform a general examination of this patient.

Salient features

- Usually men over the age of 40 years (male:female ratio is 2:1).
- Symmetrical, painless, rubbery lymph nodes.
- Liver or spleen may be palpable.

Questions

How may this patient present?

Some 25% of cases are asymptomatic; some complain of generalised malaise, weight loss and loss of appetite; others complain of bleeding.

What are causes of generalised lymphadenopathy?

- Lymphoproliferative disorders – lymphatic leukaemia, Hodgkin's disease.
- TB.
- Sarcoidosis.

■ How would you stage chronic lymphatic leukaemia?

- Stage A, no anaemia or thrombocytopenia and less than three areas of lymphoid enlargement.
- Stage B, no anaemia or thrombocytopenia, with three or more involved areas.
- Stage C, anaemia and/or thrombocytopenia, regardless of the number of areas of lymphoid enlargement.

How would you treat such a patient?

- Specific treatment may not be indicated until stage B or C.

- Stage B and C will require specific and supportive therapy, i.e. correction of anaemia and folic acid deficiency, and correction of bone marrow infiltration initially with prednisolone and oxymetholone and subsequently with chemotherapeutic agents such as chlorambucil. Combination chemotherapy (CHOP regime) and radiotherapy have also been used. Intravenous immunoglobulin reduces the incidence of infection.

Case 171 | Crohn's Disease

Instruction

These patients have chronic diarrhoea.
Examine this patient's face.
Examine this patient's abdomen (Patients 1 and 2).
Comment on this patient's perianal area.

Salient features

- Mass in the right iliac fossa (*Patient 1*).
- Multiple fistulous openings in the right iliac fossa (*Patient 2*).
- Swollen lips (*Patient 3*).
- Multiple perianal fistulous tracts (*Patient 4*).

- In all four patients, examine for the following:
    In the mouth for aphthous ulcers.
    Uveitis.
    Anaemia.
    Arthropathy.
    Skin lesions – erythema nodosum, pyoderma gangrenosum.
    Liver disease.

Questions

What investigations would you do?

- Sigmoidoscopy and biopsy.
- Small bowel study.
- Barium enema.
- Colonoscopy.

Mention some complications.

- Iritis.
- Arthritis.
- Erythema nodosum.
- Pyoderma gangrenosum.

■ Mention some associated diseases.

- Ankylosing spondylitis (HLA B27 positive).
- Sacroiliitis.
- Cholangitis, hepatitis, cirrhosis.

Mention some ocular features of Crohn's disease.

Eye lesions are seen in about 5% of cases.
- Common: conjunctivitis, anterior uveitis.
- Rare: scleritis, keratitis, keratoconjuctivitis sicca, choroiditis, retinal vasculitis, optic neuritis and orbital pseudotumour.

How would you treat Crohn's disease?

- Sulphasalazine for colonic disease.
- Steroids for small bowel disease.
- Metronidazole for perianal disease and fistulas; 6-mercaptopurine may be useful in severe cases.
- Surgery is reserved for intestinal fistulas and intestinal obstruction that does not respond to medical management.

Burrill Bernard Crohn (b. 1884) was a physician in Mount Sinai Hospital, New York; he described this condition in 1932 and pointed out the nontuberculous aetiology.

References

Crohn, BB, Ginzburg, L & Oppenheimer, GD (1932) Regional ileitis: a pathologic and clinical entity. *JAMA* **99**: 1323–1329.

Kirsner, JB & Shorter, RG (1982) Recent developments in nonspecific inflammatory bowel disease. *N Engl J Med* **306:** 775, 783.
Petrilli, EA, McKinley, M & Troncale, FJ (1984) Ocular manifestations of inflammatory bowel disease. *Clin Neurol Ophthalmol* **4:** 3.
Podolsky, DK (1991) Inflammatory bowel disease. *N Engl J Med* **325:** 1008.

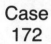

Case 172 Dysphagia

Instruction

Patient 1 has difficulty in swallowing; would you like to ask him or her a few questions?

Salient features

• Ask about the following:
  The duration of symptoms.
  Whether the difficulty is for swallowing liquids or solids or both.
  Nasal regurgitation.
  Whether or not the patient coughs on swallowing.
  The level at which the food sticks (suprasternal notch or midsternal).
  Associated heart burn.
  Weight loss.

Instruction

Patient 2 has difficulty in swallowing, would you like to examine him or her?

Salient features

- Examine as follows:
  Mouth for ulcers, thrush and pallor; check the gag reflex.
  Neck for lymph glands and goitres.
  For scleroderma.
- Tell the examiner that you would like to investigate for underlying neurological defects (evidence of stroke, motor neuron disease, myasthenia gravis).

Questions

Mention a few causes of dysphagia.

- Benign oesophageal stricture.
- Carcinoma of the oesophagus.
- Peptic ulcer of the oesophagus.
- Achalasia cardia.
- Pharyngeal pouch.
- Retrosternal goitre, bulber palsy, myasthenia gravis, Plummer–Vinson syndrome (Paterson–Kelly syndrome).

How would you investigate such a patient?

- FBC, ESR.
- Barium swallow.
- Gastroscopy.

HS Plummer and PP Vinson, both physicians at the Mayo Clinic, Rochester, Minnesota.
DR Paterson and A Brown Kelly both British ENT surgeons.

Case 173	Diarrhoea

Instruction

Patient 1 has diarrhoea; would you like to ask him or her a few questions?

Salient features

- Ask about the following:
  Onset.
  Duration of diarrhoea.
  Frequency.
  Whether or not it is nocturnal.
  Blood (seen in ulcerative colitis, shigellosis, diverticulitis, carcinoma of the colon) and muscus in the stools; blood on the toilet paper.
  Nature of the stools (pale and bulky and difficult to flush away in steatorrhoea).
  Associated pain in the abdomen.
  Appetite.
  Weight loss.
  Associated vomiting and nausea.
  Drug ingestion (including antibiotics and laxatives).
  Foreign travel.

Instruction

Patient 2 has diarrhoea, would you like to examine him or her?

Salient features

- Look for the following signs.
  Anaemia.
  Clubbing.
  Aphthous ulcers.
  Abdominal tenderness, abdominal masses.

- Tell the examiner that you would like to do a rectal examination and check for faecal occult blood.

Questions

What do you understand by the term 'diarrhoea'?

It implies passing of increased amounts of loose stool (more than 300 g per day).

How would you investigate a patient with diarrhoea?

- FBC, ESR.
- Serum albumin.
- Sigmoidoscopy.
- Stool chart, stool cultures, faecal fat.
- Barium enema, small bowel barium studies.

What are the mechanisms of diarrhoea?

- Osmotic diarrhoea: the mucosa of the gut acts as a semipermeable membrane; the diarrhoea stops when the patient fasts. Examples: diarrhoea due to magnesium sulphate, lactulose, malabsorptive states.
- Secretory diarrhoea: there is active secretion of intestinal fluid. Example: *Escherichia coli* diarrhoea.
- Inflammatory diarrhoea: there is mucosal damage. Examples: shigellosis, ulcerative colitis.
- Increased gut motility, e.g. irritable bowel syndrome.

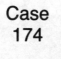

| Case 174 | Marfan's Syndrome |

Instruction

Look at this patient.
Examine this patient's heart.

Salient features

- Disproportionately long limbs as compared to the trunk – the arm span will exceed the height.

- Examine the following:
  Hands, for spidery fingers or arachnodactyly (confirm by asking the patient to clench his or her thumb in his or her fist, and put his or her fingers around his or her wrist), hypermobile joints.
  Eyes, for iridodonesis or ectopia lentis (subluxation upwards) – the patient may be wearing thick spectacles; blue sclera.
  Palate, for high arched palate.
  Skin, for small papules in the neck (Miescher's elastoma).
  Chest, for pectus excavatum, cystic lung disease.
  Heart, for mitral valve prolapse, aortic aneurysm, aortic regurgitation.
  Spine, for kyphosis.

- Tell the examiner that you would like to proceed as follows:
  Take a family history (autosomal dominant).
  Measure the ratio of upper segment to lower segment; this will be less than 0.85 (the upper segment is from the crown to the symphysis, whilst the lower segment is from the symphysis pubis to the ground).

- Remember that each patient should be referred for ophthalmic examination, annual echocardiography and genetic counselling to maximise the preventive potential in this disease.

Questions

What is your differential diagnosis?

Homocystinuria (recessively inherited inborn error of amino acid metabolism due to a deficiency of cystathionine β-synthetase), in which the skeletal features are similar.

How would you differentiate the two?

In homocystinuria the lens is dislocated downwards and there is homocystine in the urine.

What is the common cause of mortality in Marfan's syndrome?

Cardiovascular complications cause 95% of deaths in such patients and reduce mean life expectancy by 40%.

What are the ocular features of Marfan's syndrome?

- Subluxation of lens.
- Small and spherical lens.
- Glaucoma.
- Hypoplasia of dilator pupillae, making pupillary dilatation difficult.
- Flat cornea.
- Myopia.
- Retinal detachment.

What are the complications of pregnancy in women with Marfan's syndrome?

- Early premature abortions.
- Risk of maternal death from aortic dissection.

Is there a gene implicated in causing Marfan's syndrome?

The Marfan syndrome appears to be caused by mutations in a single fibrillin gene on chromosome 15.

EJA Marfan (1858–1942), French paediatrician, wrote his paper in 1896. He was appointed Foundation Professor of Hygiene at the Clinic of Infantile diseases in Paris in 1914.
Victor McKusick, contemporary Professor of Medicine at Johns Hopkins whose chief interest is genetics.

References

Editorial (1990) Fibrillin and Marfan's syndrome: a real clue. *Lancet* **336**: 973.
Pyeritz, RE (1981) Maternal and foetal complications of pregnancy in the Marfan's disease. *Am J Med* **71**: 784.
Pyeritz, RE (1991) Marfan syndrome. *N Engl J Med* **323**: 987–989.
Pyeritz, RE & McKusick, VA (1972) The Marfan syndrome. *N Engl J Med* **300**: 772–777.
Tsipouras, P, Del-Mastro, R, Safarazi, M et al (1992) Genetic linkage of the Marfan syndrome, ectopia lentis, and congenital contractural arachnodactyly to fibrillin genes on chromosomes 15 and 5. *N Engl J Med* **326**: 905.

Case 175	Nephrotic Syndrome

Instruction

Look at this patient.

Salient features

- Generalised oedema – puffiness of face, pitting leg oedema, hands.
- Look at the nails for ridges of hypoproteinaemia.
- Comment on the pallor.
- Tell the examiner that you would like to: examine the urine for protein and sugar.

Questions

What do you understand by the term 'nephrotic syndrome'?

It consists of albuminuria (more than 3.5 g per day) and hypoalbuminaemia, accompanied by generalised oedema, hyperlipidaemia and lipiduria.

What causes this syndrome?

- Glomerular disease: minimal change glomerulonephritis, membranous glomerulonephritis, proliferative glomerulonephritis.
- Systemic causes: diabetes mellitus, SLE, amyloidosis, drugs (captopril, gold, pencillamine, street heroin), Hodgkin's disease, syphilis, malaria, HIV, hepatitis B.

How would you investigate these patients?

- 24-hour urinary protein, creatinine clearance, urine electrophoresis.
- FBC, ESR.
- U&E, creatinine, albumin, cholesterol.
- DNA antibody, antinuclear factor, complement levels.
- Renal biopsy.

What complications may such a patient suffer?

- Thromboembolic events, including renal vein thrombosis and deep vein thrombosis.
- Protein malnutrition.
- Accelerated atherosclerosis.
- Infection.

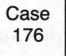

Case 176   Uraemia

Instruction

Patient 1: would you like to ask this uraemic patient some questions?

Salient features

Ask about the following:

- Anorexia, nausea, vomiting and hiccups.
- Fatigue.
- Polyuria, nocturia, dysuria, haematuria, difficulty in passing urine.
- Swelling of the face and feet.
- Shortness of breath (due to secondary left ventricular failure).
- Itching.
- Drug history, in particular NSAIDs, tetracycline.
- History of diabetes, hypertension, recurrent urinary tract infections.
- Family history of renal disease, in particular polycystic kidneys.
- Tell the examiner that you would like to take a history of impotence.

Instruction

Patient 2: would you like to examine this uraemic patient?

Salient features

- Examine the nails (for Lindsay's 'half-and-half' nails where the proximal portion is whitish while the distal portion is brownish red; the lunula is usually obscured).
- Comment on the lemon tinge of the skin, the pallor and scratch marks. Rarely, there may be 'uraemic' frost.
- Examine the arms for haemodialysis fistula.
- Comment on the vascular shunts, if any.
- Comment on hyperventilation of Kussmaul's respiration secondary to metabolic acidosis.
- Examine the abdomen for palpable kidneys (hydronephrosis, polycystic kidneys) and palpable bladder.
- Check for pitting leg oedema.

- Tell the examiner that you would like to proceed as follows:
  Check the blood pressure (hypertension, hypotension).
  Look for pericardial friction rub.
  Look for evidence of peripheral neuropathy.
  Do a rectal examination.
  Examine the urine for sugar, albumin, specific gravity, microscopy.

Questions

How would you investigate patients with renal failure?

- Urine: glucose, microscopy, specific gravity, creatinine clearance, 24-hour urinary protein.
- Blood: FBC, ESR.
- Serum: urea, electrolytes, creatinine, protein, calcium, phosphate, uric acid.
- Ultrasound of the abdomen for kidneys, bladder.
- Special investigations: pyelography, protein electrophoresis, kidney biopsy.

What do you understand by the term 'azotaemia'?

Azotaemia indicates an elevated urea and creatinine without symptoms.

What do you understand by the term 'uraemia'?

Uraemia implies a deterioration of renal function associated with symptoms.

What are the common causes of chronic renal failure?

- Glomerulonephritis.
- Diabetes mellitus.
- Hypertensive nephropathy.
- Pyelonephritis.
- Polycystic kidney disease.
- Analgesic nephropathy.

Mention a few drugs that you would avoid in renal failure.

Aminoglycosides, frusemide with cephalosporins, potassium salts, tetracycline.

What are the consequences of chronic renal failure?

- Metabolic: sodium imbalance, hyperkalaemia, metabolic acidosis, hyperuricaemia, hypocalcaemia, hypermagnesaemia, hyperphosphotaemia.
- Cardiovascular: cardiac failure, hypertension, accelerated atherosclerosis, pericarditis.
- Haematological: anaemia, clotting disorders, leucocyte abnormalities.
- Skin: itching, hyperpigmentation, bruising.
- CNS: encephalopathy, peripheral neuropathy.
- Gastrointestinal: anorexia, nausea, vomiting, peptic ulcer, diarrhoea.
- Endocrine: vitamin D disorders, secondary hyperparathyroidism, impotence, amenorrhoea, glucose intolerance.

When would you consider dialysis?

- Hyperkalaemia (potassium concentration greater than $7 \, \text{mmol} \, l^{-1}$).
- Bicarbonate less than $12 \, \text{mmol} \, l^{-1}$.
- Urea greater than $20 \, \text{mmol} \, l^{-1}$.
- Creatinine greater than $500 \, \mu\text{mol} \, l^{-1}$.

PG Lindsay, American physician.

Case 177 — Abdominal Aortic Aneurysm

Instruction

Examine this patient's abdomen.
This patient presented with low back pain; examine his or her abdomen.

Salient features

- Large expansile pulsation along the course of the abdominal aorta.
- Auscultate for bruit over the aneurysm and over the femoral pulses.
- Examine all peripheral pulses.

- Tell the examiner that you would like to check the following:
    Urine for sugar.
    Blood pressure.
    Serum cholestrol.
    History of smoking.

Questions

Which investigation would you do to confirm your diagnosis?

- Ultrasound of the abdomen – simple, cheap and accurate screening test.
- Large aneurysms would require angiography.

■ How would you manage an abdominal aneurysm?

Aortic aneurysms more than 5 cm carry a high risk of rupture and hence should be referred to the vascular surgeon for surgery. Smaller aneurysms must be followed up and they enlarge at the rate of about 0.5 cm a year.

What is the prognosis of such aneurysms?

Mortality rate for elective surgery is less than 5%, whereas the mortality of a ruptured aneurysm is nearly 90%.

References

Fowkes, FGC, MacIntyre, CCA & Ruckley, CV (1989) Increasing incidence of aortic aneurysms in England and Wales. *Br Med J* **298:** 33–35.

Greenhlagh, RM (1990) Prognosis of abdominal aortic aneurysm. *Br Med J* **301:** 136.

Nevitt, MP, Ballard, DJ & Hallet, JW (1989) Prognosis of abdominal aortic aneurysms. *N Engl J Med* **321:** 1009–1014.

Taylor, PR & Wolfe, JHN (1991) ABC of vascular diseases: treating aortic aneurysms. *Br Med J* **303:** 1127.

Case 178 Paget's Disease

Instruction

Examine this patient's face.
Examine this patient's legs.

Salient features

Face:

- Comment on the hearing aid, if any. Test hearing and determine if the deafness is a conduction defect (due to involvement of the ossicle) or neural (due to compression of the eighth nerve).
- Typical appearance of the skull and increased skull diameter (more than 55 cm is abnormal).
- Tell the examiner that you would like to examine the fundus for optic atrophy or angioid streaks.

Neck:

- Look for platybasia.
- Raised JVP (cardiac failure in Paget's is due to hyperdynamic circulation).

Spine:

- Deformity of the spine – kyphosis; auscultate over the vertebral bodies for bruits.

Legs:

- Comment on the anterior bowing of the tibia and the lateral bowing of the femur.
- Feel the bone for warmth.
- Tell the examiner that you would like to examine the joints for osteoarthritis (limitation of hip movement, in particular abduction, and fixed flexion deformity of the knees).

- Tell the examiner that you would like to proceed as follows:
  Do a urine analysis (high incidence of renal stone).
  Measure the patient's height (for serial follow-up).
  Compare the patient's appearance with previous photographs.
  Ask the patient whether or not there is an increase in hat size.

Questions

What are complications of Paget's disease?

- Diminished mobility.
- Fractures.
- Cord compression due to basilar invagination.
- Root lesions due to vertebral damage.
- Hypercalcaemia.
- High output cardiac failure.
- Sarcomatous changes are seen in less than 2% of cases.

Mention the neurological complications of Paget's disease.

- Headache.
- Fits.
- Platybasia.
- Hydrocephalus.
- Cerebellar signs.
- Cranial nerve palsies.
- Cord compression.

What are the mechanisms of hearing loss in such patients?

- It is usually due to the disease process involving the ossicles.
- Less commonly it is due to progressive closure of the skull foramina compressing the eighth cranial nerve.

What is the basic defect in bone metabolism?

Increased osteoclastic activity resulting in bone resorption and increased osteoblastic activity.

What are the radiological manifestations of this disease?

- Skull: 'honeycomb' appearance with underlying osteoporosis circumscripta, 'cotton wool' appearance.
- Pelvis: thickening of the iliopectineal line 'brim sign', enlargement of ischial and pubic bones.
- Long bones: increased trabeculation.
- Vertebra: sclerotic margins giving a 'picture frame' appearance.
- Remember that bone scan is more sensitive than X-ray in determining the extent of disease.

What is the prevalence of Paget's disease?

The exact prevalence is not known but several reports indicate a 3% prevalence in patients over the age of 40 years and increases with age to reach a maximum of 10% by the ninth decade. Males predominate by a ratio of about 2:1.

What factors have been implicated in the aetiology of Paget's disease?

- Slow virus infection – measles syncytial virus.
- Genetic factors have been described in Italy.

What are the biochemical features of this disease?

- Serum calcium is normal (except in prolonged immobilisation or malignancy).
- Increased bone serum alkaline phosphatase (indicates increased osteoblastic activity).
- Increased urinary hydroxyproline secretion (indicates increased bone resorption).

Which drug is commonly used in the treatment of this disease?

Diphosphonates (they inhibit bone resorption).

To which patients would you offer therapy?

Treatment is offered to patients with any of the following symptoms:
    Agonizing bone pain.
    Severe deformity.
    Hypercalcaemia.
    Cardiac failure.

Sir James Paget (1814–1899), Surgeon, St Bartholomew's Hospital, London. He also described Paget's disease of the nipple (carcinoma involving the areola and the nipple), Paget's disease of the skin (skin cancer involving the apocrine glands) and Paget–Schroetter syndrome (venous thrombosis of the axillary veins, of unknown cause).

References

Paget, J (1877) On a form of chronic inflammation of bones (osteitis deformans). *Med Chir Trans* **60**: 37.

| Case 179 | Parotid Enlargement |

Instruction

Look at this patient's face

Salient features

- Bilateral parotid enlargement.
- Look for the following conditions:
    Dry mouth.
    Lupus pernio.
    Rheumatoid arthritis.
- Tell the examiner that you would like to know whether the patient has gritty eyes or dry mouth.

Questions

What are the causes of painless bilateral parotid enlargement?

- Sarcoidosis.
- Sjögrens syndrome or keratoconjuctivitis sicca.
- Lymphoma and leukaemia.

How would you test objectively for dry eyes?

Schirmer's test: filter paper is hooked over the lower eyelid; in normal people at least 15 mm is wet in 5 minutes and a value of less than 5 mm is seen in sicca syndrome.

■ **What do you know about keratoconjuctivitis sicca?**

It is a condition characterised by decreased production of tears by lacrimal glands.

Mention a few causes of keratoconjuctivitis sicca.

● Primary keratoconjuctivitis sicca is common and characterised by the involvement of the lacrimal gland alone.
● Primary Sjögren's syndrome is an autoimmune disorder which is usually positive for rheumatoid factor, antinuclear antibodies and hypergammaglobulinaemia. Less frequently, autoantibodies to DNA, salivary gland, smooth muscle and gastric parietal cells are present. There may be associated dry mouth and bronchial epithelium, and the vagina may also be affected.
● Secondary Sjögren's syndrome is the presence of keratoconjuctivitis sicca in association with a systemic disorder such as the following:
    Rheumatoid arthritis.
    Psoriatic arthritis.
    Connective tissue disorder.
    Sarcoidosis.
    Crohn's disease.

How would you manage such patients?

● Artificial tears (e.g. hypromellose) are instilled frequently for dry eyes.
● Artificial saliva for dry mouth.

OWA Schirmer (1864–1917), German ophthalmologist.

Case 180 | Superior Vena Caval Obstruction

Instruction

Look at this patient.

Salient features

- Tortuous, visible and dilated veins on the chest wall and neck.
- The neck veins are nonpulsatile.
- The face may be plethoric and suffused. The patient may be short of breath.

- Look for signs of Horner's syndrome and for radiation marks.
- Tell the examiner that you would like to examine for signs of bronchogenic carcinoma, i.e. clubbing, tar staining, lymph nodes, chest signs.

Questions

What symptoms might the patient have?

- Shortness of breath.
- Dysphagia.
- Blackouts.
- Facial oedema.

What are the causes of superior vena caval obstruction?

- Bronchogenic carcinoma is the commonest cause.
- Lymphoma – in young adults.
- Other causes:
    Aortic aneurysm.
    Mediastinal goitre
    Mediastinal fibrosis.

■ How would you manage this patient?

This condition is a medical emergency and an urgent CT scan of the chest should be requested. Emergency treatment consists of the following:

- Intravenous frusemide to relieve the oedematous component of vena caval compression.
- Intravenous cyclophosphamide.
- Mediastinal irradiation within 24 hours.

References

Sculier, JP & Field, R (1985) Superior vena cava obstruction syndrome. Recommendation for management. *Cancer Treat Rev* **12:** 209.

Case 181	Glass Eye

Instruction

Look at this patient's fundus.
Examine this patient's eyes.
Check this patient's vision or visual fields.

Salient features

- Glass eye which is obvious.
- The patient is blind on the affected side.

- Tell the examiner that you would like to take a history of trauma.

Note. Suspect malignant melanoma if asked to examine the abdomen and the liver is palpable (due to metastases).

Case 182	Turner's Syndrome

Instruction

Look at this patient.

Salient features

- Webbing of the neck in a female patient.
- Abnormal angulation of both elbows – increased carrying angle (cubitus valgus).
- Dwarfism.
- Shield-shaped chest – nipples are widely separated.

- Tell the examiner that you would like to proceed as follows:
    Check for radiofemoral delay (coarctation of the aorta).
    Examine genitalia for infantilism.

Questions

What constitutes a web?

Either a fan-like fold of skin extending from the shoulder to neck, or an abnormal splaying out of the trapezius.

What is the chromosomal defect?

It is due to the absence of one of the X chromosomes.

Henry H Turner (b. 1892), an American endocrinologist, described the condition in 1938.

Case 183 Yellow Nail Syndrome

Instruction

Examine this patient's hands.

Salient features

- Yellowish discoloration of the nails.
- Tell the examiner that you would like to proceed as follows:
  Examine the chest (for pleural effusion, bronchiectasis).
  Examine the legs for lymphoedema.
  Ask about past history of sinusitis.

Questions

What is the aetiology?

The aetiology is obscure and is thought to be related to lymphatic hypoplasia.

How would you manage such patients?

Symptomatically. No treatment is known to influence the condition.

References

Runyon, BA, Forker, EL & Sopko, JA (1979) Pleural fluid kinetics in a patient with primary lymphoedema, pleural effusions and yellow nails. *Am Rev Respir Dis* **119:** 821.

Case 184	Osteogenesis Imperfecta

Instruction

Look at this patient's eyes.

Salient features

- Blue sclera.
- Look for the following signs:
  Hearing loss due to otosclerosis.
  Signs of old fractures.
  Defective dentin formation in the teeth.
  Kyphosis and scoliosis.
  Joint hypermobility.
  Hernias.
- Tell the examiner that you would like to ask some questions:
  About previous fractures.
  Whether or not it runs in the family.

Questions

Why is the sclera blue?

Because the choroid pigment is visible.

Mention other conditions in which the sclera is blue.

- Marfan's syndrome.
- Ehlers–Danlos syndrome.

■ What is the inheritance?

Usually autosomal dominant although some cases may be autosomal recessive.

What are clinical types?

- Osteogenesis imperfecta congenital, in which fractures occur *in utero* and skeletal abnormalities are present at birth.

- Osteogenesis imperfecta tarda, in which fractures and deformities occur after birth.

References

Editorial (1986) Molecular genetics and osteogenesis imperfecta. *Lancet* 2: 496.

Case 185	Down's Syndrome

Instruction

Look at this patient.

Salient features

- Collapse of the bridge of the nose.
- Low-set ears.
- Epicanthic folds.

- Look at the iris for Brushfield's spots, i.e. yellow speckles seen in young children.
- Tell the examiner that you would like to proceed as follows:
  Examine the hands for simian palmar crease and short inward curving of the little finger.
  Examine the heart for murmur of mitral regurgitation (endocardial cushion defects), and ASD (ostium primum type).
  Check MSQ.
  Formal IQ testing.
  Ask the mother at what age she delivered the child.

Questions

What complications can be seen in such patients?

- Increased incidence of leukaemia.
- Presenile dementia of Alzheimer type.
- Atlantoaxial subluxation.

Mention two chromosomal abnormalities seen in this condition.

- Trisomy 21.
- Mosaicism (46XY/47, XY, +21).

What are the underlying genetic mechanisms?

- Nondysjunction.
- *De novo* translocation.
- Familial translocation.

JLH Langdon Down (1828–1896) wrote an article in *Clinical Lectures and Reports of The London Infirmary* (now the Royal London Hospital) in 1866 entitled 'The ethnic classification of idiots'.
T Brushfield (1858–1937), British physician.

Case 186	Late Congenital Syphilis

Instruction

Look at this patient.

Salient features

- Collapsed bridge of nose (saddle nose).
- Corneal opacity (interstitial keratitis).
- Rhagades (linear scars at the angles of the mouth).

- Peg-shaped incisors (Hutchinson's teeth).
- Perforation of the palate.
- Frontal bossing.

- Tell the examiner that you would like to proceed as follows:
  Check for deafness (nerve deafness).
  Look at the shins for sabre tibia.
  Look for Clutton's joints (bilateral knee effusions).
  Look at the fundus for optic atrophy.

Questions

What is Hutchinson's triad?

- Interstitial keratitis.
- Deafness.
- Typical dental changes, i.e. peg-shaped incisors (Hutchinson's teeth).

What are the ocular features of congenital syphilis?

- Interstitial keratitis.
- Retinopathy – fine pigmentation, 'salt and pepper fundus'.

Sir Jonathan Hutchinson (1828–1913) was simultaneously a surgeon at The London Hospital (now Royal London Hospital), an ophthalmologist at Moorfields Hospital and a dermatologist at Blackfriars Hospital (now closed).
H Clutton (1850–1901), English surgeon who worked at St Thomas's Hospital.

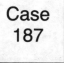

Arteriovenous Fistula

Instruction

Look at this patient's arms.

Salient features

- Hypertrophy of the affected arm.
- Prominent, dilated tortuous veins.
- Continuous thrill over the fistula; listen for continuous bruit.
- Collapsing pulse; increased pulse pressure indicating hyperdynamic circulation.

- Look for signs of cardiac failure.
- Elicit Branham's sign, i.e. slowing of the pulse on occluding the feeding vessel of the fistula.
- If the fistula is in the upper limb then perform Allen's test: the radial and ulnar arteries are occluded at the wrist and the hand is exercised; the arteries are then released one at a time to establish which is the dominant feeding vessel.
- Look for signs of chronic renal failure.

Questions

What is the aetiology of peripheral arteriovenous malformations?

- Surgical – for chronic haemodialysis in patients with renal failure.
- Post-traumatic.
- Congenital.

How are arteriovenous malformations classified?

Angiographically, as follows:

- Group 1, predominantly arterial or arteriovenous lesions: present with pain, hypertrophy of the digit or limb, deformity, distal ischaemia, venous hypertension; large lesions can cause symptoms and signs of cardiac failure.
- Group 2, lesions affecting tiny vessels including capillaries: for example, port wine stain, epistaxis in hereditary haemorrhagic telangiectasia, gastrointestinal haemorrhage with colonic dysplasia.
- Group 3, predominantly venous lesions: local oedema, pain and venous ulceration; there may be a history of trauma.

How would you manage a patient with an arteriovenous malformation?

- Referral to a vascular surgeon.
- Doppler ultrasonography.
- Angiography.

When and how is an arteriovenous malformation treated?

Arteriovenous malformations are treated when they cause discomfort, disfigurement and danger to the patient. The patient should be jointly assessed by a vascular surgeon and an interventional radiologist for embolisation. Temptation to surgically ligate the feeder vessel should be resisted as subsequent embolisation may be difficult. Complete excision of the fistula is accepted treatment in resistant cases.

EV Allen (1900–1961), Professor of Medicine at the Mayo Clinic, Rochester, Minnesota, introduced courmarin anticoagulants into clinical practice and edited one of the first comprehensive textbooks on peripheral vascular disease.
HH Branham, American surgeon in the nineteenth century.

References

Allison, DJ & Kennedy, A (1991) ABC of vascular diseases: peripheral arteriovenous malformations. *Br Med J* **303:** 1191–1194.

Case 188	Carotid Artery Aneurysm

Instruction

Examine this patient's neck.

Salient features

- Pulsatile swelling along the course of the carotids, usually unilateral (the swelling may be firm) and at the base of the neck.

- Auscultate over the mass for a bruit.
- Look for Horner's syndrome.

- Tell the examiner that you would like to proceed as follows:
    Examine all peripheral pulses.
    Examine the heart and blood pressure.

Questions

How would you manage this patient?

    All patients must be referred to a vascular surgeon.
    Check urine for sugar.
    Serum lipids.
    Intravenous carotid digital subtraction angiography.

Case 189	Retro-orbital Tumour

Instruction

Examine this patient's eyes.

Salient features

- Unilateral exophthalmos.
- Impaired extraocular movement (due to either muscle or nerve involvement).
- Chemosis, conjunctival oedema.
- Radiation marks may be present.

- Examine the visual acuity and visual fields.
    Look for pulsations over the globe.
    Palpate the orbital margin for erosion of the underlying bone.
    Auscultate over the globe for bruit.

Questions

What is your differential diagnosis?

- The commonest cause of unilateral exophthalmos is Graves' disease.
- Other causes are as follows:
  Retro-orbital tumour (primary or metastatic).
  Arteriovenous fistulas.
  Cavernous sinus thrombosis.

What investigations would you do?

- T_4, TSH, free T_3.
- Orbital ultrasound.
- Cranial CT, in particular the orbits.

How would you manage such a patient?

- Ophthalmology opinion.
- Therapy – radiation to the orbit and steroids, and surgical decompression – depending on the underlying aetiology.

What are the causes of an unilateral pulsating proptosis?

- Arteriovenous fistula between the carotid artery and cavernous sinus – stops with pressure on the artery in the neck.
- Aneurysm of the ophthalmic artery.
- Cirsoid aneurysm of the orbit.
- Vascular neoplasms in the orbit growing rapidly.

FUNDUS

Examination of the Fundus

1. Tell the patient, 'Look straight ahead with your right or left (R/L) eye while I look into your L/R eye'. (The candidate need not remove his or her own spectacles while examining the fundus.) The candidate should use his or her own R/L eye to examine the patient's R/L eye.

2. Look at the eye from a distance of at least 50 cm and check for red reflex. (The presence of a red reflex indicates that the media in front of the retina is transparent and that the retina is firmly in apposition with the underlying choroid. Red reflex may be absent when there is a lens opacity, vitreous haemorrhage or retinal detachment.)

3. Look systematically at the following:
   - The optic discs (comment on the colour, contour, cup and lamina cribrosa).
   - The macula (one to two disc diameters away from and a little below the temporal margin of the optic disc).
   - The nasal and temporal halves of the fundus.
   - The retinal vessels (remember that the retinal artery has four main branches and the normal ratio of the artery to the vein is 2:3).

Case 190	Diabetic Retinopathy

Instruction

Examine the fundus in these patients.

Salient features

You will be expected to comment on whether it is background or proliferative retinopathy. You may have a clue about underlying diabetes either from a diabetic chart or from the presence of diabetic fruit juices at the bedside.

Patient 1 has background retinopathy, caused by microvascular leakage into the retina.

- Microaneurysms, usually seen in the posterior pole temporal to the fovea.
- Dot and blot haemorrhages.
- Hard exudates.

Questions

What symptoms will this patient have?

The patient will be asymptomatic as the macula is spared.

How would you manage such a patient?

- Treat diabetes and associated hypertension.
- Annual fundal examination.

Salient features

Patient 2 has diabetic maculopathy, caused by oedema and/or hard exudates.

- Signs of background retinopathy with hard exudates or oedema of the macula.

Questions

What symptoms may the patient have?

There will be a gradual impairment of central vision, such as difficulty in reading small print or seeing road signs.

How will you manage this patient?

Nonurgent referral to an ophthalmologist for photocoagulation which will stabilise (seldom improve) visual acuity in 50% of the cases.

Salient features

Patient 3 has preproliferative retinopathy which is uncommon and is caused by retinal hypoxia.

- Cotton-wool spots.
- Venous dilatation, beading, looping or sausage-like segmentation.
- Arteriolar narrowing.
- Haemorrhages – large, dark blots.
- Intraretinal microvascular abnormalities (IRMAs).

Questions

What symptoms may this patient have?

Asymptomatic if the macula is spared.

How would you manage this patient?

Semiurgent referral to the ophthalmologist for close follow-up to enable early detection and treatment of proliferative retinopathy.

Salient features

Patient 4 has proliferative retinopathy, caused by retinal hypoxia and usually seen in insulin-dependent diabetic retinopathy.

- Neovascularisation around the disc (NVD) or away from the disc – in the early stages the vessels are bare and flat and easily missed. In later stages they are elevated and may be associated with white fibrous component.
- Presence of laser burns (in treated cases).

Questions

What symptoms may this patient have?

Asymptomatic in the absence of complications.

How would you manage this patient?

Urgent referral to an ophthalmologist for laser treatment.

What are the complications of proliferative retinopathy?

- Vitreous haemorrhage.
- Traction retinal detachment.
- Rubeosis irides.
- Rubeotic glaucoma – some of these patients can have partial restoration of vision by microsurgery called pars plana vitrectomy.

What is the prevalence of retinopathy in diabetes?

The overall prevalence is about 25%. It is 40% in insulin-dependent diabetes mellitus (IDDM) and 20% in non-insulin-dependent diabetes mellitus (NIDDM).

What is the relationship between the duration of diabetes and retinopathy?

There is a close relationship: in patients diagnosed to have diabetes before the age of 30 years the incidence of retinopathy is about 50% after 10 years and 90% after 30 years. It is unusual for retinopathy to develop within 5 years of onset of diabetes; however, 5% of NIDDMs have background retinopathy at presentation.

What associated systemic conditions worsen diabetic retinopathy?

- Pregnancy.
- Hypertension.
- Anaemia.
- Renal failure.

What is the relationship between diabetic control and retinopathy?

Good control will delay the development of retinopathy but will not prevent it.

How often would you screen diabetic patients for retinopathy?

- Non-insulin-dependent diabetics: annually.
- Insulin-dependent diabetics:

Newly diagnosed: no screening for the first 5 years.
Five to ten years from initial diagnosis: annually.
Over 10 years after initial diagnosis: every 6 months.

What is the earliest sign of retinal change in diabetes?

An increase in capillary permeability, evidenced by the leakage of dye into the vitreous humour after fluorescein injection, is the earliest sign of retinal change in diabetes mellitus.

What do you know about photocoagulation?

Photocoagulation is a technique whereby several thousand lesions are produced over a 2-week therapy using lasers. It decreases the incidence of haemorrhage or scarring in proliferative retinopathy. It is also useful in the treatment of microaneurysms, haemorrhages and oedema. Some loss of peripheral vision may be inevitable with this technique.

What surgical technique may be used for a nonresolving vitreous haemorrhage and retinal detachment?

Pars plana vitrectomy may be used but is often complicated by retinal tears, retinal detachment, glaucoma, infection, cataracts and loss of the eye.

What is the role of hypophysectomy in diabetic retinopathy?

Hypophysectomy was widely performed in the past but is no longer recommended.

Do you know of any drug which may prevent proliferative retinopathy?

Betacyclodextrin tetradecasulphate (an experimental heparin analogue) may prevent proliferative retinopathy by inhibiting angiogenesis.

MJ Williams, contemporary physician, Aberdeen, has written the biography of Professor Macleod, a British physiologist who was awarded the Nobel Prize with Banting.

References

Editorial (1989) Diabetic retinopathy. *Lancet* 1: 1113.
Merimee, TJ (1990) Diabetic retinopathy. *N Engl J Med* 322: 978–983.

Case 191	Hypertensive Retinopathy

Instruction

Examine this patient's eyes.
Examine this patient's fundus.

Salient features

- Arteriovenous nipping.
- Arteriolar narrowing.
- Macular star.
- Flame-shaped and blot haemorrhages.
- Cotton-wool exudates.
- Papilloedema may or may not be present.

- Tell the examiner that you would like to check the blood pressure.

Questions

How would you grade hypertensive retinopathy?

- Stage I, arteriolar narrowing.
- Stage II, irregular calibre of arterioles.
- Stage III, cotton-wool exudates; flame and blot haemorrhages.
- Stage IV, papilloedema.

Mention a few causes of the hypertension.

- In 90% of cases it is essential hypertension with no underlying cause and this may represent the 'normal' spread.
- In 10% of cases there is an underlying cause:

- Renal causes: renal artery stenosis, polycystic kidneys, chronic glomerulonephritis, polyarteritis nodosa, chronic pyelonephritis.
- Endocrine causes: Cushing's syndrome, Conn's syndrome, phaeochromocytoma, acromegaly, diabetes mellitus.
- Eclampsia and pre-eclamptic toxaemia of pregnancy.
- Coarctation of the aorta.

How would you investigate a patient with hypertension?

- Urine for protein, glucose, casts.
- Midstream urine for microscopy and culture.
- U&E, fasting lipids.
- CXR.
- ECG.
- Urinary cathecholamines.
- Intravenous pyelogram.
- Renal artery DSA.

How would you treat hypertension?

- Salt restriction.
- Drug therapy.
- First line:
  In women and smokers – bendrofluazide.
  In nonsmoking men – beta blocker.
- Advise the patient to stop smoking.

Sir CT Dollery, contemporary Dean, Royal Postgraduate Medical School, Hammersmith Hospital, London; his interests include clinical pharmacology, hypertension and medical education.
John Swales, contemporary Professor of Medicine, Leicester; his chief interest is hypertension.
JC Petric, contemporary Professor of Medicine and Therapeutics, Aberdeen, his interests include hypertension and cardiovascular prevention.

References

Dollery, CT, Ramalho, PS, Patterson, JW et al (1965). Retinal microemboli: experimental production of 'cottonwool' spots. *Lancet* 1: 1303.
Swales, JD (1990) First line treatment in hypertension. *Br Med J* 301: 1172.

Case 192	Papilloedema

Instruction

Examine this patient's fundus.

Salient features

- There is swelling of the optic disc (look for haemorrhages and soft exudates).

Note. Remember that the common causes are as follows:
Intracranial-space-occupying lesion.
Hypertensive retinopathy.
Benign intracranial hypertension.

Questions

What do you understand by the term 'papilloedema'?

Papilloedema is the swelling of the nerve head as seen on ophthalmo-scopy. The colour of the disc becomes redder, approximating to that of the rest of the retina; its contour becomes blurred and the cup and cribrosa are filled in.

What is the first manifestation of papilloedema?

The earliest manifestation of papilloedema is engorgement of the veins.

What is the nature of field defect in papilloedema?

Papilloedema is always associated with the enlargement of the blind spot, with a consequent diminution of visual fields and gradual loss of visual acuity, but a fair acuity may remain until papilloedema is marked.

■ Mention a few causes of papilloedema.

- Raised intracranial pressure resulting from one of the following conditions:

Impaired circulation of the CSF due to aqueduct stenosis.
Meningitis.
Subarachnoid haemorrhage.
- Cerebral oedema:
  Post head injury.
  Post cerebral anoxia.
- Metabolic causes:
  Carbon dioxide retention.
  Steroid withdrawal.
  Thyroid eye disease.
  Vitamin A intoxication.
  Lead poisoning.
- Increased protein in the CSF due to one of the following:
  Guillain–Barré syndrome.
  Spinal cord tumours.
  Any spinal block.
- Haematological and circulatory disorders:
  Central retinal vein thrombosis.
  Superior vena caval obstruction.
  Polycythaemia vera.
  Multiple myeloma.
  Macroglobinaemia.

Mention a few conditions simulating papilloedema.

- Deep optic cup:
  Nasal edge appears heaped up.
  Vessels plunge into the optic cup.
  Temporal edge is quite normal.
- Medullated nerve fibres, seen on the disc or even on the retina. The appearance is typically flared and on focusing will reveal fibres traversing the area. Field defects are due to the retinal vessels being obscured. Since these are present from birth the patient is unaware of the defect.
- Bergmeister's papilla, in which there is whitish elevation of the centre of the disc with venous and arterial sheathing. It is common and seen in all ages. There is an equal sex and racial incidence.
- Pseudopapilloedema, i.e. congenitally elevated discs secondary to hyaloid tissue (drüsen) or hyperopia.

Note. Elevation or swelling on the optic disc occurs in the following conditions:
Papilloedema.
Papillitis.
Drüsen.
Infiltration of the nerve head by malignant cells.

What do you know about Foster Kennedy syndrome?

Unilateral papilloedema with or without 'secondary' optic atrophy on the other side suggests a tumour of the opposite olfactory lobe or orbital surface of the frontal lobe or of the pituitary body.

What do you understand by the term 'papillitis'?

Papillitis is the term used to describe disc swelling associated with optic neuritis; it is accompanied by early visual loss. Causes are as follows:
- Demyelination of the optic nerve.
- Inflammation.
- Degeneration (Leber's optic atrophy).
- Vascular disorders of the nerve head.
- Malignant cell infiltration.

How do you differentiate papillitis from papilloedema?

Papillitis	Papilloedema
Usually unilateral	Usually bilateral
Visual acuity is considerably reduced in relation to degree of swelling of the disc	Visual acuity only slightly reduced until late stages
Visual field defect is usually central, particularly for red and green	Peripheral constriction or enlargement of blind spot
Marcus Gunn pupil may be present	Marcus Gunn pupil is absent
Eye movements may be painful	Eye movements are never painful

Note. A Marcus Gunn pupil is one which shows better constriction to an indirect response than to direct light.

What are the stages of papilloedema?

- Stage I, increase in venous calibre and tortuosity.
- Stage II, optic cup becomes pinker and less distinct, the vessels seeming to disappear suddenly on the surface of the disc.
- Stage III, blurring of the discs on the nasal side. (**Note.** In many normal discs the nasal edge is less distinct and one of the most frequent false-positive signs is questionable blurring of nasal disc margins.)
- Stage IV, the whole disc becomes suffused and slightly elevated. The margins may disappear and the vessels seem to emerge from a mushy swelling. The optic cup is filled and there are haemorrhages around the disc.

Foster Kennedy (1884–1952) was born in Belfast. He was Professor of Neurology at Cornell University. He described his syndrome in 1923.

References

Sanders, MD & Sennehenn, RH (1980) Differential diagnosis of optic disc oedema. *Trans Ophthalmol* Soc UK **100:** 123–131.

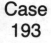 **Optic Atrophy**

Case
193

Instruction

Examine this patient's eyes.
Examine this patient's fundus.

Salient features

- Pale disc with sharp margins.
- Intact consensual light reflex but impaired direct light reflex – Marcus Gunn pupillary response (seen in asymmetrical involvement of the two eyes).
- Central scotoma on testing of visual fields.

Note. Remember that multiple sclerosis is the commonest cause and tell the examiner that you would like to look for cerebellar signs.

Questions

What is your diagnosis?

The differential diagnosis is as follows:
- Demyelinating disorders (multiple sclerosis).
- Optic nerve compression by tumour or aneurysm.
- Glaucoma.

- Toxins: methanol, tobacco, lead, arsenical poisoning.
- Ischaemic, including central retinal artery occlusion due to thromboembolism, temporal arteritis, idiopathic acute ischaemic optic neuropathy, syphilis.
- Hereditary disorders: Friedreich's ataxia, Leber's optic atrophy (sex-linked, seen in young males).
- Paget's disease.
- Vitamin B_{12} deficiency.
- Secondary to retinitis pigmentosa.

■ What is the difference between primary and secondary optic atrophy?

- Primary optic atrophy is one which has not been preceded by papilloedema.
- Secondary optic atrophy follows papilloedema.

Primary	Secondary
White and flat with clear-cut edges	Greyish-white, edges are indistinct
Visible lamina cribrosa	Cup filled and lamina cribrosa not visible
Arteries and veins normal	Arteries thinner than normal Veins may be dilated
Capillaries decreased in number (less than seven) – Kestenbaum's sign	Capillaries decreased in number

What is consecutive optic atrophy?

Consecutive optic atrophy is a controversial term and is best avoided. Some use it as an equivalent or alternative for what has been described above as secondary optic atrophy, but others use the term to indicate an atrophy complicating choroiditis or, rarely, a retinitis such as Tay–Sachs disease or retinitis pigmentosa.

What is glaucomatous optic atrophy?

Glaucomatous optic atrophy denotes loss of disc substance, referred to as increased cupping.

How would you investigate a patient with optic neuropathy?

- FBC, ESR.
- Blood glucose.
- Serology for syphilis.
- Vitamins B_{12} and B_1 levels.

- Skull X-ray of pituitary fossa, optic foramina and sinuses, or CT scan of brain and orbit.
- ECG.
- Pattern-stimulated visual evoked responses.
- Electroretinography.

R Marcus Gunn (1850–1909), Scottish ophthalmologist who worked at Moorfields Eye Hospital, London.
T von Leber (1840–1917), Professor of Ophthalmology at the University of Heidelberg, Germany.
W Tay (1843–1927), British ophthalmologist, Moorfields Eye Hospital, London.
BP Sachs (1858–1944), German neuropsychiatrist who worked in New York. He described this condition independent of Tay.

Case 194 — Retinal Vein Thrombosis

Instruction

Examine this patient's eyes.
Examine this patient's fundus.

Salient features

Patient 1 has central retinal vein occlusion:

- Multiple retinal and preretinal haemorrhages surround the optic nerve head. There is marked dilatation and tortuosity of the veins, hyperaemia or oedema of the nerve head and soft exudates – 'blood and thunder' appearance.
- Visual acuity is only slightly reduced.

Patient 2 has branch vein occlusions:

- These occur just distal to the arteriovenous crossing. The superior temporal vein is most commonly involved. Haemorrhages are seen surrounding the occluded vein.

- May cause a quadrantic field defect.
- Visual prognosis is good if the haemorrhages do not extend to the macula with accompanying macular oedema.
- Tell the examiner that you would like to check for the following conditions:
    Diabetes (urine sugar).
    Hypertension.
    Chronic simple glaucoma.
    Hyperviscosity syndromes – Waldenström's macroglobulinaemia, multiple myeloma.

Questions

How would you manage such eyes?

- Treat the underlying condition.
- Regular follow-up by the ophthalmologist as secondary neovascularisation is a common sequela and may need laser therapy.

JC Waldenström (b.1906), Professor of Medicine, Uppsala University, Sweden.

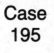

Case 195   Retinitis Pigmentosa

Instruction

Examine this patient's fundus.
Examine this patient's eyes.

Salient features

- Peripheral retina shows perivascular 'bone spicule pigmentation' and arteriolar narrowing. The retinal veins (never the arteries) often have a sheath of pigment for part of their course. The pigment spots which lie near the retinal vessels are seen to be anterior to them, so that they hide the course of the vessels. (In this respect they differ from the pigment around spots of choroidal atrophy in which the retinal vessels can be traced over the spots.)

• Optic disc is pale.
• Maculopathy which is atrophic or cystoid.

• Look for polydactyly in the hands and feet (Laurence–Moon–Biedl syndrome).
• Comment on white walking aid (if any) used by the legally blind.

Questions

What is the prognosis in retinitis pigmentosa?

Most patients are legally blind by the age of 40, with central field less than 20 degrees in diameter. Almost all patients lose central vision by the seventh decade.

What do you know about retinitis pigmentosa?

Retinitis pigmentosa is a slow degenerative disease of the retina. It occurs in both eyes, begins in early childhood and often results in loss of sight by middle or advanced age. The degeneration primarily affects the rods and cones, in particular the rods.

How may it present?

It may present with defective vision at dusk (night blindness) which may occur several years before the pigment is visible in the retina.

■ Mention a few systemic disorders associated with retinitis pigmentosa.

• Laurence–Moon–Biedl–Bardet syndrome, which is a recessively inheritied disorder characterised by mental handicap, polydactyly, syndactyly, hypogonadism and obesity.
• Bassen–Kornzweig syndrome (abetalipoproteinaemia), characterised by fat malabsorption, abetalipoproteinaemia, acanthocytosis and spinocerebellar ataxia.
• Refsum's disease (phytanic acid storge disease), an autosomal disorder characterised by hypertrophic peripheral neuropathy, deafness, ichthyosis, cerebellar ataxia, elevated CSF protein in the absence of pleocytosis.
• Kearns–Sayre syndrome, a triad of retinitis pigmentosa, progressive external ophthalmoplegia and heart block.

- Usher's disease, a recessively inherited disorder characterised by congenital, nonprogressive, sensorineural deafness.
- Friedreich's ataxia (see page 119).

What ocular conditions are associated with retinitis pigmentosa?

- Open-angle glaucoma.
- Posterior subcapsular cataracts.
- Myopia.
- Keratoconus.

What is secondary retinitis pigmentosa?

Secondary retinitis pigmentosa is a sequel to an inflammatory retinitis. It is often ophthalmoscopically indistinguishable from the primary condition, the electroretinogram and electro-oculogram response is slightly subnormal unless the condition is far advanced. (In the primary type the response is markedly subnormal to electroretinogram and electro-oculogram.)

What is retinitis pigmentosa sine pigmento?

A variety of retinitis pigmentosa but without visible pigmentation of the retina.

What is inverse retinitis pigmentosa?

Bone corpuscles are visible in the perifoveal area while the retinal periphery is normal.

JZ Laurence (1830–1874), English ophthalmologist.
RC Moon (1844–1914), US ophthalmologist.
A Biedl (1869–1933), Czech physician.
G Bardet (b.1885), French physician.
FA Bassen (b.1903), physician, and AL Kornzweig (b.1900), ophthalmologist, Mt Sinai Hospital, New York.
S Refsum, Norwegian physician.

References

Cogan, DG, Rodrigues, M, Chu, FC et al (1984) Ocular abnormalities in abetalipoproteinemia. *Ophthalmology* **91:** 991.
Dryja, TP, McGhee, TL, Hahn, LB et al (1990) Mutations within the rhodopsin gene in patients with autosomal dominant retinitis pigmentosa. *N Engl J Med* **323:** 1502.
Fishman, GA, Kumar, A & Joseph, ME (1983) Usher's syndrome. *Arch Ophthalmol* **101:** 1367.
McKechnie, NM, King, M & Lee, WR (1985) Retinal pathology in Kearns–Sayre syndrome. *Br J Ophthalmol* **69:** 63.

Case 196	Subhyaloid Haemorrhage

Instruction

Examine this patient's fundus.

Salient features

- A large, solitary subhyaloid haemorrhage (there may be no fluid level if the patient is lying flat).
- There may be associated retinal haemorrhage.
- 20% may have mild papilloedema.

When the subhyaloid (preretinal) haemorrhage extends into the vitreous humour it is called Terson's syndrome.

Questions

What is the commonest cause of a subhyaloid haemorrhage?

Subarachnoid haemorrhage.

What are the other causes of haemorrhages into the vitreous?

- Local injury.
- Blood diseases.
- Hypertension.
- Diabetes.
- Idiopathic.

Mention some causes for neck stiffness.

- Subarachnoid haemorrhage.
- Meningitis.
- Posterior fossa tumours.
- Local neck pathology such as cervical spondylosis.

What are causes of deterioration in a patient with subarachnoid haemorrhage?

- Rebleeds.

- Cerebral infarction due to reflex vasospasm of cerebral vessels (hence the rationale to use nimodipine).
- Secondary hydrocephalus.

How would you investigate such a patient?

CT head scan, and if this rules out intracranial hypertension then a lumbar puncture to diagnose minor leaks.

References

Ostergaard, JR (1990) Warning leak in subarachnoid haemorrhage. *Br Med J* **301**: 190.

Case 197	Old Choroiditis

Instruction

Examine this patient's fundus.

Salient features

- Old or inactive retinochoroiditis appears as white, well-defined areas of chorioretinal atrophy with pigmented edges (due to proliferation of retinal pigment epithelium).
- The retinal blood vessels pass over the lesions undisturbed.

Questions

What may be the aetiology?

- Reactivation of congenital toxoplasmosis.
- Cytomegalovirus infections.

- AIDS.
- Sarcoidosis.
- TB.
- Syphilis.
- Behçet's disease.

What is the prognosis?

Prognosis varies according to the underlying aetiology. It is poor if the fovea is involved.

What does the presence of pigment on fundoscopy indicate?

The presence of a chronic lesion of the retina or the choroid.

In which other conditions is retinal pigment seen?

- Normally – racial (tigroid fundus).
- Retinitis pigmentosa.
- Malignant melanoma.

H Behçet (1889–1948), Professor of Dermatology in Turkey, described this syndrome in 1937 based on three patients he observed between 1924 and 1936.

Case 198	Cholesterol Embolus in the Fundus

Instruction

Examine this patient's fundus.

Salient features

- Presence of a cholesterol embolus (Hollenhorst plaques) in one of the branches of the retinal artery.

Questions

What are the complications of such an embolus?

Retinal artery occlusion causing field defects or loss of vision.

Where is the likely origin of this embolus?

The most likely origin is an atherosclerotic plaque in the carotid circulation.

What do you understand by the term 'amaurosis'?

Amaurosis means blindness from any cause.

What do you understand by the term 'amblyopia'?

Amblyopia means impaired vision not due to refractive error or ocular disease.

What do you understand by the term 'amaurosis fugax'?

Amaurosis fugax is a retinal artery TIA which manifests with a painless, unilateral loss of vision that usually lasts for a few minutes.

How would you manage this patient?

- Aspirin.
- Ophthalmology opinion.
- Ultrasound of carotid arteries.
- Advise the patient to stop smoking.
- Control of hypertension.
- Carotid angiogram with a view to performing a carotid endarterectomy.

What is the effect of cholesterol crystals?

Cholesterol crystals rarely cause significant obstruction to the retinal arterioles.

What manoeuvre would you use to make the cholesterol crystals more apparent?

Mild lateral pressure on the globe may make the presence of unobtrusive crystals clearly visible when the retinal arterioles pulsate.

How would you manage an acute occlusion of the retinal artery?

- Lie the patient in the supine position to ensure adequate circulation.
- Intermittent ocular massage is applied for 15 minutes to dislodge the emboli, lower intraocular pressure and improve circulation.

- Intravenous acetazolamide to lower the intraocular pressure.
- Inhalation of a mixture of 5% carbon dioxide and 95% oxygen.
- Anterior chamber paracentesis.

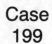

Case 199   Vitreous Opacities

Instruction

Examine this patient's fundus.

Salient features

- Small, white opacities which are present in front of the retinal vessels.
- The patient may complain of diplopia (monocular diplopia).

- Tell the examiner that you would like to proceed as follows:
  Test for monocular diplopia.
  Check urine for sugar.
  Check the blood pressure.

Questions

What are causes of diplopia?

- Myasthenia gravis.
- Third, fourth or sixth cranial nerve palsy.
- Weakness of the extraocular muscles.

What are the other causes of monocular diplopia?

- Opacities in the lens.
- Corneal opacities.
- Retinal detachment.

Case 200	Myelinated Nerve Fibres

Instruction

Examine this patient's fundus.

Salient features

- White, streaky patches which extend from the disc and terminate peripherally in a feather-like pattern. It may cover the retinal vessels.

Questions

What is the pathology?

Occasionally, the myelination of the optic nerve does not stop at the lamina cribrosa but extends onto nerve fibres surrounding the optic disc. This condition is a benign congenital abnormality known as medullated or myelinated nerve fibres. It terminates peripherally in a feather-like margin with fine striations from the course of the nerve-fibre layer.

INDEX